THE
HIGH-PERFORMING
MEDICAL PRACTICE

Workflow, Practice Finances, and Patient-Centric Care

OWEN J. DAHL, MBA, LFACHE, CHBC

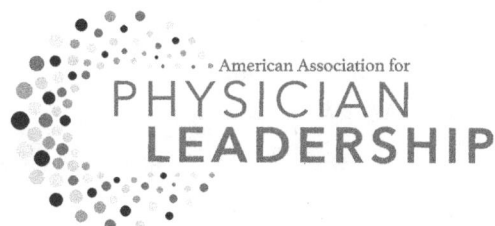

American Association for
**PHYSICIAN
LEADERSHIP**

Published by **American Association for Physician Leadership, Inc.**
PO Box 96503 | BMB 97493 | Washington, DC 20090-6503

Website: www.physicianleaders.org

AAPL books are available at special quantity discounts to use as premiums and sales promotions, or for use in corporate training programs. For more information, please write to Special Sales at journal@physicianleaders.org

This publication is designed to provide general information and is sold with the understanding that neither the author nor the publisher is engaged in rendering legal, accounting, ethical, or clinical advice. If legal or other expert advice is required, the services of a competent professional person should be sought.

13   8 7 6 5 4 3 2 1

Copyedited, typeset, indexed, and printed in the United States of America

PUBLISHER
Nancy Collins

EDITORIAL ASSISTANT
Jennifer Weiss

DESIGN & LAYOUT
Carter Publishing Studio

COPYEDITOR
Emily Collins

ACKNOWLEDGMENTS

This book is dedicated to my wife, Noela, and to my children and grandchildren. Additional thanks go to Nancy Collins and the entire publishing team at Greenbranch Publishing. I also want to thank Ken Hertz and my many others colleagues who have shared their experiences with me. They have allowed me to learn from them and to better focus on applying business principles in the medical practice. After all, taking care of patients is what medical practice is all about.

TABLE OF CONTENTS

ABOUT THE AUTHOR

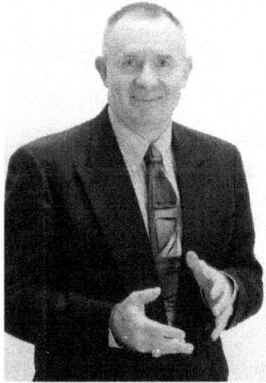

Owen J. Dahl, MBA, LFACHE, CHBC, LSSMBB, has been active in healthcare management for almost 50 years. He received his bachelor's degree from Concordia College, Moorhead, MN, where he was a member of the first graduating class in the hospital administration program. He received his Master's degree from the University of Northern Colorado and has done additional study at NOVA Southeastern in Ft. Lauderdale, FL. He spent more than a decade as a hospital administrator in various facilities in South Dakota. He also served in the United States Air Force and the Army National Guard.

His move to New Orleans in 1983 brought a major career change. He started a practice management and billing company, which grew to manage 65 physicians in 11 different practices. In 1993 he advanced to Fellow in the American College of Health Care Executives with a paper on Total Quality Management and its application to the medical practice. Hurricane Katrina brought about another change that has lead to his current efforts as an author, consultant, public speaker, and adjunct professor. He has worked with Loyola University in New Orleans, the University of New Orleans, Louisiana State University School of Medicine, the University of Houston – Clear Lake on physician practice management programs.

Throughout his career Mr. Dahl has maintained a passion to seek to improve the delivery of patient care through training and education. He developed the first certification program for the Professional Association of Health Care Office Managers (PAHCOM) and the certification program for the National Society of Certified Health Care Business Consultants (NSCHBC). Currently, an independent consultant with an affiliation with the Medical Group Management Association (MGMA) he has developed training programs in various "belt" levels in Lean Six Sigma and the application to today's medical practice.

He is the author of *Think Business! Medical Practice Quality, Efficiency, Profits, Second Edition*. He is co-author to *Lean Six Sigma for the Medical Practice: Improving Profitability by Improving Processes*; *Integrating Behavioral Health into the Medical Home: A Rapid Improvement Guide*; and *Disaster Planning for the Medical Practice*, all published by Greenbranch Publishing (www.greenbranch.com). He is also co-author of *Benchmarking Success: The Essential Guide to Group Practices, Second Edition*.

Mr. Dahl is married with three children and two grandchildren. He currently resides in The Woodlands, TX. Contact Owen Dahl at www.owendahlconsulting.com.

Introduction and
The Value Star Concept

In examining the US healthcare system from different perspectives, does the system work? Are there changes to be made? Where should these changes take place? In Washington or at the State Capitol? At the hospital or healthcare system? In the physician office?

What can we control? Where can we have the greatest influence? Remember what the physician practice is all about – providing patient care by meeting the patient's expectations.

The intent of this book is to challenge you and your healthcare practice colleagues to define a process to focus on the patient, including their population health. We will concentrate on the things you can control in your practice. We will also discuss the factors that have the greatest opportunity for transformation in the healthcare practice.

Today's healthcare system is a complex network. The number of participants, with their own objectives, contrasts the healthcare networks found in many other countries. The overriding objectives that have been espoused by government programs including the transition to value-based, outcome-based delivery options. These programs focus on population health which is defined as the health outcomes of a group of individuals.

Table 1 shows that the United States ranks far ahead many other countries in costs of care, based on 2013 statistics.[1]

As of 2016, the percentage of Gross Domestic Product (GDP) had risen to 17.9% which represents $3.3 Trillion on healthcare and the per capita expenditure to $10,348.[2]

TABLE 1. Healthcare Spending Percentages GDP

	% GDP	Per Capita	Phys per 1000	Visits per Phys
US	17.1%	$9,086	2.6	4.0
France	11.6%	$4,361	3.1	6.4
Sweden	11.5%	$5,153	4.0	2.9
German	11.2%	$4,920	4.1	9.9
Netherlands	11.1%	$5,131		6.2
UK	8.8%	$3,364		

Many other statistics are included such as mentioned infant mortality, average life expectancy, and the like. Again, the US ranks mid-to-low in these statistics. There are pockets of success but there are many excuses why we have not had an impact on the statistics. TW²ADI, is an acronym for "The Way We've Always Done It" which is unacceptable today.

PATIENT OUTCOMES

Figure 1 illustrates the four major factors influencing health outcomes for patients and for population health.[3]

1. Individual Health Behaviors
2. Social and Economic Factors
3. Physical Environment
4. Clinical Care including Access and Quality of Care

Individual behaviors, social and environmental factors, and the physical environment make up 80% of expected health outcomes. The other 20% relate to what healthcare practices do daily, including clinical access to care and quality of care.

Given this, it seems as if we have little opportunity to impact patient outcomes if we only concentrate on clinical care. What do we do about the other factors? Many of the electronic medical record programs, the Medicare Access and CHIP Reauthorization Act (MACRA) program, and the like are attempting to help the clinician address these factors.

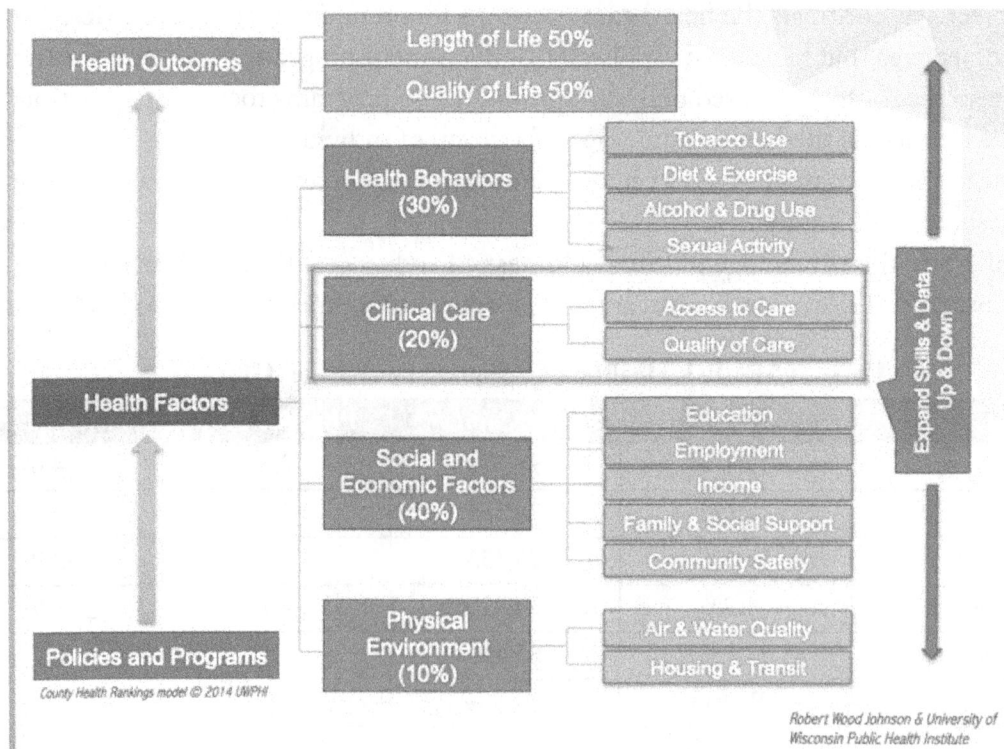

FIGURE 1. Major Factors Influencing Health Outcomes

TRENDS

A recent trend has been toward consolidation of physician practices either merging together, becoming part of a hospital, healthcare system, or merging with payers. Recent data suggests that less than 50% of all physician practices are now part of these models rather than independent practices.[4]

There is also a movement to create Patient Center Medical Homes (PCMH) or variations of the same for specialty practices. Healthcare systems and some practices are developing Accountable Care Organizations, or ACOs.

1. A PCMH or, The Medical Home is defined as a model or philosophy of primary care that is patient-centered, comprehensive, team-based, coordinated, accessible, and focused on quality and safety. There are five features of the medical home: patient-centered, comprehensive, coordinated, accessible, and committed to quality and safety.

There are many attempts beyond the PCMH to achieve the above points and with the passage of the Affordable Care Act (ACA), the main emphasis has been on Accountable Care Organizations. These are defined by Centers for Medicare & Medicaid Services (CMS) as applying to Medicare but an ACO can serve and work with multiple private payers as well.

2. Accountable Care Organizations (ACOs) are groups of doctors, hospitals, and other health care providers, who come together voluntarily to give coordinated and high-quality care to their Medicare patients.

    The goal of coordinated care is to ensure that patients, especially the chronically ill, get the right care at the right time, while avoiding unnecessary duplication of services and preventing medical errors.

Organizations have come together under the Medicare Shared Savings Program and to date the 350+ ACOs have saved Medicare substantial dollars. Savings are shared by the government and the ACO members. These ACOs have expanded to cover non-Medicare patients through various third-party payer arrangements.

This book is offered as a challenge to everyone who provides healthcare to our citizens and population. The answers to the questions in the initial paragraph are, "yes, we can change, and we need to change." And it starts with the point of contact for most patients, the physician's office.

I hope to encourage thoughts that result in a transition or even a transformation of today's medical practice into a new and improved way of doing things. As we know, "every patient is different," and "every healthcare practice is different". While this may be true there are still many aspects of every practice that can be improved; can benefit from transformation.

Let's examine the patient experience, from the patient's perspective and from the healthcare practice's perspective.

THE PATIENT EXPERIENCE: REALITY

1. <u>The Patient Experience…from the Healthcare Practice Perspective. New Patient and Established Patient</u>

a. New Patient

Appointment phone call:
- "Good Morning, Dr. Smith's office, this is Owen, how may I help you?"
- Patient is requesting to see Dr. Jones, an associate.
- Reason for the visit given.
- Offer date, day, and possible time. Patient accepts.
- Obtain date of birth, phone number, address, and appropriate demographic information.
- Obtain insurance information.
- Referring doctor if any, or other doctors seen.
- After 10 minutes on the phone, confirm appointment date and time.
- End with the request for the patient to go online to complete patient information and to please arrive 20 minutes early to the appointment.
- Call is complete.

Prior to the visit:
- Patient account set up is completed.
- Insurance coverage is verified.
- Appointment reminder process scheduled to begin.

Patient arrives at the office:
- Patient signs in and finds a seat.
- Patient is called to the desk, given a clipboard (or tablet) with instructions to complete all pages, sign where noted and asked to return to the desk.
- Thank you to patient, material is reviewed, ensuring business info is captured.
- Co-pay, deductible, etc. explained and collected as noted in the financial policy that was included in the packet the patient received.
- Notify the back-office patient has arrived; provide whatever clinical information received.

Patient is called back to begin the clinical process:
- Vital signs are taken, reason for visit noted, documentation complete. Notes show that patient is ready to be seen by provider.
- Patient seen, chart updated.
- Orders written (or verbally given) related to results of findings from the visit.

- Action taken recorded in the system, patient informed via script, ancillary services needed, etc.
- Patient escorted to check out.
- Exam room is straightened out and prepared for next patient.

At check out:
- Next appointment scheduled.
- Balance due collected. Fees for ancillary services or deposit for surgery collected. Patient cannot leave until financial matters are clear and understood.
- "Thank you for choosing our practice for your medical needs."

After the visit:
- At some point, documentation is completed, if necessary, by provider and staff.
- Appointments for ancillary services, surgery, admission, or whatever is necessary completed.

b. Established Patient

Prior to visit:
- Reminder system operational.

At visit:
- Patient is greeted, and payment is requested, thank you and please be seated, you will be called back soon.
- Patient is summoned by name, greeted, and escorted back to the triage area.
- Vitals taken and noted in chart.
- Update, from a clinical perspective, is recorded.
- Patient is escorted to exam room.
- Provider enters, examines the patient and determines next course of treatment.
- Medical assistant reviews orders and discusses with patient.
- Patient is escorted to check out, follow-up appointment or other activity occurs.
- "Thank you for choosing our practice for your medical needs."

After the visit:
- At some point, documentation is completed, if necessary, by provider and staff.
- Appointments for ancillary services, surgery, admission, or whatever is necessary completed.

And so, it goes. The same procedures each day for new patient visits and established patient visits. Prior to closing for the day, rooms are checked, supplies are stocked, and rooms are prepped for the morning.

Is that all there is?

No, there is more. It is all about perspective. Here is the same procedure, from the patient perspective.

2. The Patient Experience…from the Patient Perspective. New Patient and Established Patient.

a. New Patient

Prior to visit:

- Patient talks to friends and/or researches physicians and practices on the Web.
- Patient makes the phone call.
- Phone rings. "Dr. Smith's office, our menu has changed so please pay attention. If this is an emergency, hang up and call 911, if this is a doctor's office or pharmacy please press 1, if you want to schedule an appointment, press 2, etc….."
- Patient pushes 2 and is told to hold. The call volume is heavy and so we will be with you shortly. A recorded commercial plays on a loop in the background. "Please continue to hold your call is important to us."
- Phone is answered, and the registration process begins. Name please, reason for call, discussion of available appointment times, patient recites all demographic data, provides insurance numbers. Patient finds calendar, makes sure appointment time is available and notes time. Patient is referred to Web site to print and/or electronically complete several forms, which will save time on day of appointment.
- Two days prior to appointment, patient receives email reminder of the visit. Later that same day, patient receives a text regarding the same. The day before the appointment, patient receives a computer-generated call reminding patient of appointment – press 1 to confirm or press 2 to cancel. As a new patient all reminders ask that the patient arrives 20 minutes early to complete the registration process.
- The other option is to go online and do all of the above without human interaction.

Patient arrives at the office:

- Staff busy. Patient records name and time of arrival on the sign in sheet. Notes doctor to see and checks off new patient status. Patient takes seat in waiting room.
- Staff member calls patient to the desk and asks patient to complete more forms; something was missed while doing the forms online. Staff member asks for payment, patient provides credit card information. Patient told receipt will be emailed as it is impossible to print receipt in the office.
- After a 20-minute wait from the appointment time (not the 20-minute early arrival time), the medical assistant calls patient back and asks about weight and height. MA asks patient to sit down and extend left arm for blood pressure. Temperature is also taken. Patient doesn't like the result of the BP and asks that the BP is taken

again. MA takes again, and the results are more in line with what the patient expects. MA asks why patient is presenting and makes notes in the medical record. Asks questions as to why patient is here and notes in the record.

- Patient is escorted back to exam room, sits on exam table and is told the doctor will be in shortly. Interesting exam room, lots of signs and charts to read on the walls. The patient reads them all.
- Physician enters the exam room, wearing a white lab coat. Patient and physician have a very thorough visit with good exam, questions are answered, and the patient feels comfortable. Patient and physician develop a good game plan and patient stays in room until the MA comes back in.
- The MA comes in and the plan is discussed. MA will schedule tests and she asks the patient to schedule the next appointment and MA will also follow-up with the patient.
- Patient forgets to mention to the physician that he would like a refill on a medication that he had from a previous doctor.
- Patient is escorted to check out.

b. *Established Patient*

Patient arrives at the office:
- After three appointment reminders, which the patient thinks are excessive and unnecessary, the patient plans the day to ensure on-time arrival to the office.
- Patient signs in and takes a seat, the receptionist calls the patient up to the desk. Patient makes co-payment with a credit card.
- Patient sits and waits. Patient is happy the office has a Wi-Fi connection, so patient can use a tablet for the 35-minute wait. The patient is upset as he sees other patients being escorted back before he is – and those patients arrived later than he did. Why?
- The MA calls the patient back, asks about weight and height, takes blood pressure, temperature, etc. Asks the patient if there are any issues since the last visit and notes that patient is back to review test results.
- Patient is escorted to exam room where patient waits for another 15 minutes.
- The doctor enters and seems upset. She says one of the test results is not yet available and she's not sure what happened. She leaves the room to find out. It turns out that the results have not been received yet, the test was done too close to this return visit and results will not be known for two more days.
- The patient and physician have a shortened discussion and patient is told to wait for the MA to assist.
- The MA enters and escorts patient to the checkout area where patient sets up another appointment four days later that week.

Prior to patient's next visit:
- Patient has a sudden pain and calls the office to see physician availability.
- The receptionist indicates that the doctor is out and there is no provider available. Patient indicated that he thinks he needs to be seen. Since an appointment is already set up, patient is told to wait.
- This doesn't work for the patient, who then goes to the emergency room.

This is not a scenario that is too dramatic; it could be worse. But the big question is the difference between the perspective of what happens from the healthcare office staff members vs. the perspective of the patient.

SOME COMMENTS ON POPULATION HEALTH

Of course, there are many other questions that could be asked about the patient's treatment, his wellness, his financial situation, and his environment. We will explore different options in the chapters in this book. Again, we will concentrate on what can be done in the healthcare practice to improve care. Further, what about the obligation the practice must consider—not only to the needs of one patient but the needs of similar patients? Is there anything that can or should be done for fellow employees or others in the community?

Today's disjointed healthcare delivery model continues to evolve with many efforts to create a more fluid model. In attempting to understand the big picture, Table 2 illustrates a care continuum model coupled with potential models for payment for services along the steps of the continuum.

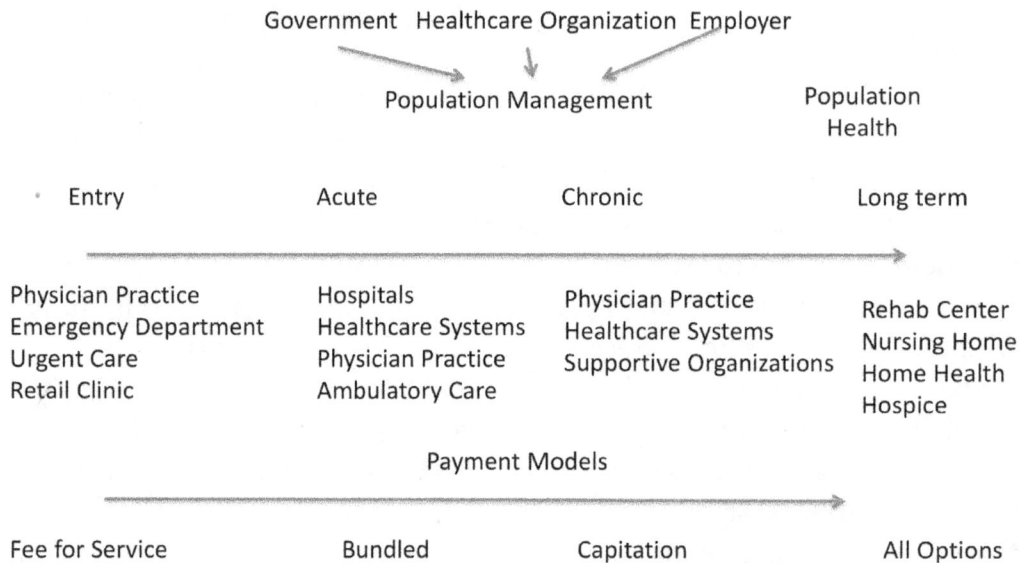

	Government	Healthcare Organization	Employer	
	Population Management			Population Health
	Entry	Acute	Chronic	Long term
	Physician Practice Emergency Department Urgent Care Retail Clinic	Hospitals Healthcare Systems Physician Practice Ambulatory Care	Physician Practice Healthcare Systems Supportive Organizations	Rehab Center Nursing Home Home Health Hospice
			Payment Models	
	Fee for Service	Bundled	Capitation	All Options

TABLE 2. Care Continuum and Payment Models

The Institute for Healthcare Improvement, The Institute of Medicine, the Affordable Care Act, and many other sources refer to the, "Triple Aim." This term refers to the simultaneous pursuit of exploring the patient experience of care, improving the health of populations, and reducing the per capita cost of healthcare. Many variations exist but we will explore this with the basic terminology of quality, access, and cost. Any effort to improve the healthcare delivery system in the United States must consider these three key aspects.

This has lead to a few concepts which encourage a focus on population health, and patient-centered care. The evolution of the PCMH and ACO has occurred as officials continue to identify the most effective delivery models.

In Table 2 we look at the many moving parts and assemble into a continuum of care, which applies, to all our citizens. If we accept population health as a goal, the first real step is to identify the concept of population management and what goes into that, which is the overriding theme of the Table 2. We start with the idea there are three main sources of input. Government relates to several items starting with the policies set by the Food and Drug Administration and other agencies related to diet and nutrition.

Next are healthcare organizations. This role will be addressed further. Next are employers who purchase health insurance and programs to incentivize good health. They can and do play a significant role.

On the top far right is the idea of population health; the key role is the individual and how they deal with their own health. The objective is for population management to help the individual achieve and maintain a healthy life style which is key in reducing healthcare costs.

The care continuum is in the center of the figure. Starting with the **entry** point and moving to the right, a patient enters the system through various options noted. The most frequent entrance is through the physician practice. The entry may very based upon need, location, payment options, etc. The entry point may be the concluding point in any spell of illness, e.g., a small laceration or cold. Treatment at the point of entry may be sufficient to resolve the issue presented.

The **acute** phase is where major treatments occur. This could be intensive care or surgery or infusion for infectious disease or cancer care. The key point here is that once the patient enters they system and they require additional care there are options available for **chronic** or **long-term** care. These episodes will vary by length and resources necessary to meet the needs of the patient.

The patient with a chronic disease is situated at the most expensive point in the care continuum. Individuals who receive acute treatment may or may not need chronic treatments. According to the National Council on Aging, the top 10 chronic conditions for Medicare patients are:[5]
1. Hypertension
2. High Cholesterol
3. Arthritis

4. Ischemic Heart Disease
5. Diabetes
6. Chronic Kidney Disease
7. Heart Failure
8. Depression
9. Alzheimer's Disease
10. Chronic Obstructive Pulmonary Disease (COPD)

Younger population includes obesity with its impact on Type 2 Diabetes. Not listed is cancer, which many now include as a chronic disease.

Last in the continuum is the long-term perspective, which is critical because 10,000 citizens are turning 65 each day.[6] Aging causes a significant increase in this area of need!

The bottom portion of Table 2 shows optional payment models. The current trend is to move from pay-for-volume to pay-for-value, V4V. Value-based payments from government and virtually all other payer sources shifts from the fee-for-service model to an outcomes-based model. Government programs are pushing this shift through its pay for reporting options, incentives for electronic reporting, and the development of coordinating care delivery models, e.g., ACOs.

Based on an outline cited by Clayton Christensen, et.al, in their book *The Innovators Prescription*, (McGraw-Hill, 2009) there may be a benefit from three or more different payment approaches. As noted under the entry stage, fee-for-service may be very appropriate. This is for that initial contact and may only require that one visit. Whether or not co-payments are necessary is not the point. It may be the easiest way to handle these transactions. The Current Procedural Terminology, CPT®, model and existing practice management systems work very well.

The more acute needs may best be handled with a bundled payment approach. This relates to the need to coordinate care with several providers, physician to facility to equipment to technology. A single payment based upon all services required for a diagnosis has been developed for joint replacements and other treatment needs and will continue to evolve. This requires different organizations to join forces (or one in the case of Geisinger, Kaiser Permanente and others) and a fair distribution of all funds to the appropriate provider.

The chronic disease segment may be not be as easy. Currently, there are at least two overriding models. There are evidence-or rules-based needs such as for diabetes. For example, it has been well established that a quarterly visit with an A1C lab test, annual foot and eye exam form the base of care. This approach can be paid via capitation or some variation of that model to control costs and to incentivize monitoring and compliance.

For diseases such as Amyotrophic Lateral Sclerosis (ALS), this area is not so well defined or is there approved evidence-based approaches. The number of patients per disease type are neither great nor is there enough research. Payments for these types may be in any one or combination of the three noted.

Long-term care will depend on the diagnosis and condition of the patient. Step down units, rehab centers, and the like may be paid on a bundled base. Home health may be paid on a fee-for-service or a modified bundled payment approach.

THE VALUE STAR CONCEPT

The Value Star Concept (Figure 2) is designed as a roadmap for every healthcare practice. Practices should follow this roadmap with the intent of improving patient care – not just for those patients served directly but for transforming the practice in the community. The Value Star concept will lead us through the chapters in this book.

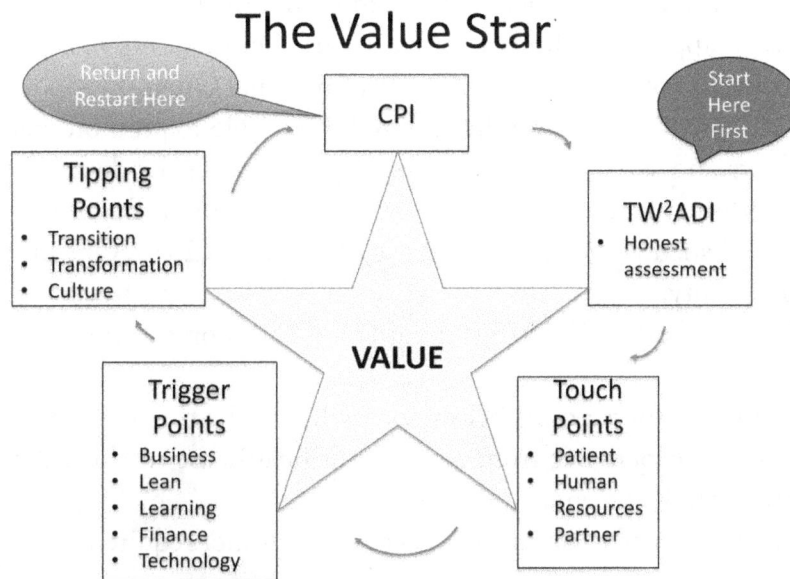

FIGURE 2. The Value Star Concept

The first point of the Value Star, on the right, suggests starting with an **honest assessment** of the state of the practice. Defining the current state by asking questions, utilizing tools addressed in Chapter 6 and identifying appropriate metrics will provide a baseline from which to measure the success of the forthcoming transition program.

The second point of the Value Star comprise the **touch points**. Touch points will be chapters two through four. These will consider the patient-centered approach to identify patient expectations through various sources, patient compliance with care plans, and employee engagement. The third point of the star focuses on **tipping points**. The tipping points focus on the tasks at hand from the learning organization to partnership in the care continuum to management and leadership to reimbursement and to technology to efficiency/effectiveness.

We will proceed to the fourth point of the Value Star which are **the trigger points**. These are the items triggering the need to transition (change), transform, and to revise the culture of the organization to clarify its role in achieving true population health. All the points of the star then lead to the fifth point—that of **continuous process improvement, or CPI**.

It is not enough to make one or a series of transitions at one time, rather it is important to adapt a culture that says we can always improve. "The Way We've Always Done It" TW2ADI is no longer acceptable as we all need to improve care for each patient and for the community that we serve.

QUALITY PRINCIPLES

It has always been clear to me that healthcare should learn and adopt other business concepts from other successful industries. There have been many times when I've encountered new and exciting ideas to apply in healthcare only to hear, "Oh that! We've been doing that for years!" from members of other industries. The International Organization for Standardization, ISO, with 162-member countries has worked since 1946 to promote standards to assist in creating products and services that are consistent and meet the demands of customers. ISO is a non-governmental, independent body based in Geneva. Beginning in 1987 standards have been published with periodic updates, the latest in 2015. One of the major areas of emphasis is on quality.

The ISO 9000:2015 and 9001:2015 standards are based on seven quality management principles.[7]

In considering each of these points below, you will find the theme of this book. Application of knowledge and experience from outside our healthcare world will help open your eyes to an improved model of care.

1. Customer focus – satisfaction surveys, meeting customer requirements, and managing relationships.
2. Leadership – vision and mission, values, trust and recognizing role of employees.
3. Engagement of people – utilize people's abilities, enable learning and sharing, and open discussion of issues and problems.
4. Process approach – activities are processes, interacting between departments, and look for process improvement opportunities.
5. Improvement – improve performance and capabilities, empower employees to make those improvements.
6. Evidence based decision making – accurate and reliable data, analytical approach to decision making based upon appropriate available data.
7. Relationship management – appropriate suppliers, optimal resource, short and long term, accept expertise of others, plan and work with partners.

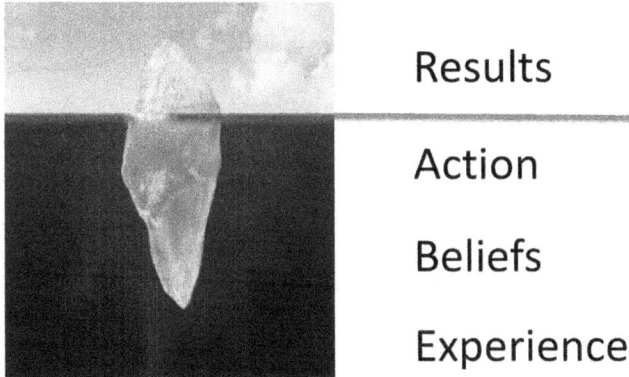

Results

Action

Beliefs

Experience

FIGURE 3. Most Activity is Below the Surface

In their book on culture and change, Connors and Smith (Penguin 2011) identified a "results pyramid" which suggests that the results of any effort are based upon the experiences of the individual.[8] These experiences lead to what they believe the behavior or actions that they or others take in the organization. Scharmer and Kaufer (Berrett-Koehler, 2013) use the model of an iceberg to address similar concepts (Figure 3).[9]

The concept here is that as you review your practice, revise your operation and seek to improve care provided to the patients served, most of the activity is below sea level, underneath, unseen. It is this activity that produces results, whether good or bad, intended or unintended. It is this activity that we seek to identify and to provide concepts and tools from which you can seek to improve your overall results.

Putting these two approaches together gives us the image of an iceberg with results clearly known but the actions taken to achieve those results are not clearly observed, understood, or even measured.

We will set the framework for an honest assessment of your practice in the Chapter 1 followed by three sections that will identify touch points, tipping points, and trigger points. These questions will provide a framework which you can use to make the transition necessary to survive and thrive in today's ever-changing market place.

Let's get started.

REFERENCES

1. The Commonwealth Fund. Healthcare Spending as a Percentage of GDP 1980-2013. October 8, 2015; https://www.commonwealthfund.org/chart/2015/health-care-spending-percentage-gdp-1980-2013. Accessed December 1, 2018.

2. AMA Wire. Growth in Health Spending Slows in Post-ACA Era. May 3, 2018; https://wire.ama-assn.org/ama-news/growth-health-spending-slows-post-aca-era. Accessed December 1, 2018.

3. Health Catalyst. Population Health Management: Systems and Success. https://www.healthcatalyst.com/population-health/ Accessed December 1, 2018.

4. AMA Wire. For First Time, Physician Practice Owners are Not the Majority. May 31, 2017; https://wire.ama-assn.org/practice-management/first-time-physician-practice-owners-are-not-majority. Accessed December 1. 2018.

5. Medicare.com. Common Health Concerns for Seniors. January 29, 2018; https://medicare.com/health/common-health-concerns-for-seniors/ Accessed December 1, 2018.

6. Yahoo Finance. 10,000 Boomers Turn 65 Every Day. Can Medicare and Social Security Handle It? May 9, 2017;.https://finance.yahoo.com/news/10-000-boomers-turn-65-111500689.html. Accessed December 1. 2018.

7. ASQ.org. What is the ISO 9000 Standard Series? http://asq.org/learn-about-quality/iso-9000/overview/overview.html. Accessed December 1, 2018

8. Conners R, Smith T. *Change the Culture Change the Game*, New York, NY: Penguin Group; 2011.

9. Scharmer O, Kaufer, K. *Leading from the Emerging Future: From Ego-System to Eco-System Economies*, San Francisco, CA: Berrett-Koehler; 2013.

Chapter 1

An Honest Assessment of Your Healthcare Practice

The big question for every provider is how to survive, or rather thrive, in the uncertainty of today's healthcare environment. This book is not intended to answer questions about mergers with other practices, or purchases by hospitals and other entities. Instead, this book intends to encourage a look at the basic business model of YOUR practice environment.

In this chapter, we will review some of the basic questions and explore some possible answers. Throughout the next few pages, we will look at your business, and discuss aspects that we believe are key to long-term survival for your practice.

In the Introduction, we cited the possibility of different payment options for various sources of care on the continuum. We wish to expand this discussion to focus on the physician practice. Regardless of the specialty, it is important to consider what you are offering to the patients who seek care in your practice.

The first place to start is with the patient. There is a distinct possibility that any provider, while seeing patients in the office on any one day, will see one of four different types of patients:

- The patient seeking diagnosis or basic treatment. This could be as simple as a cold, or as complex as a serious heart ailment. In some cases immediate treatment is provided and the issue is resolved. In other cases, the need for a care plan – acute or chronic in nature - will complete that day's visit.
- The patient who has been diagnosed and is in need of more advanced treatment. In some cases, this may be in the office, but mostly in other, more appropriate settings.
- The chronic patient who has been seen before, perhaps many times in the office or other settings.
- The patient seeking a wellness exam/experience. Accepting the model of meeting the need for population health, all providers, regardless of specialty and/or training, have a role to play in addressing the patient expectation and population need.

As a provider, are you meeting the needs and providing the best treatment option for that patient in your office setting? If the practice is so busy that you only have a few minutes with each patient, are you utilizing your resources effectively? Should you even be seeing the patient for that level of care in that setting? Do you have the resources available in your setting to provide optimal care to the patient? Can you get reimbursed appropriately for meeting that patient's need?

Before we go any further, consider the payment models noted in the continuum framework. Perhaps the diagnostic visit should be fee-for-service, the treatment visit could be part of a bundled package, the chronic visit part of a capitation model, and the wellness visit part of any of the three options. Are your treatment plans geared around payment options? Do you treat patients differently if they are fee-for-service vs. one of the other options? If so, why? Are financial incentives driving these decisions, or is it the best possible option for care?

Let's look at each of the different patient phases by asking additional questions:

- The patient in need of diagnosis may need an x-ray or lab service. Do you have the capabilities in the office? If it is necessary to send out for service, is that cost effective? Is that best for the patient?

- If you have a capitation contract, is it better to refer out from a cost point of view, or should you purchase the appropriate equipment? Have you considered that even though it may not be a direct return on investment, would it be cheaper to provide the service in the office rather than refer out?

- In the wellness exam, do you pre-order diagnostic procedures so you can review results, or do you make the patient come back for a "sickness" visit to review results?

This may seem like a lot of questions, but in order to honestly assess your practice, you need to do a true detailed review of everything.

Let's now look at your practice in greater detail. An honest assessment of how well you are doing - what is good and what is bad - is a great place to start. The long-proven format of a SWOT analysis helps to identify these factors. SWOT (For Strengths, Weaknesses, Opportunities, and Threats) features a review of what you consider to be your strengths and weaknesses internally. The opportunities and threats relate to your position in the local market. It is critical to be honest and complete. The following four tables will guide your review.

TABLE 1-1. SWOT Strengths — Internal

• Many service lines	• Portfolio management
• Broad market coverage	• New-venture management expertise
• Service competence	• Appropriate management styles
• Good marketing skills	• Appropriate organizational structure
• Good supply system	• Appropriate control systems
• R&D skills & leadership	• Ability to manage strategic change
• Information systems	• Well developed corporate strategy
• Human resources	• Good financial management
• Brand name reputation	

TABLE 1-2. SWOT Weaknesses — Internal

- Obsolete, narrow service line
- Rising production costs
- Decline in R&D innovations
- Poor marketing plan
- Poor supply system
- Loss of patient good will
- Inadequate information systems
- Inadequate human resources
- Loss of brand name
- Growth without direction
- Bad portfolio management
- Loss of corporate direction
- Infighting among departments
- Loss of corporate control
- Inappropriate organizational structure
- High conflict & politics
- Poor financial management

TABLE 1-3. SWOT Opportunities — Environmental

- Expand core business
- Exploit new market segments
- Widen service range
- Extend differentiation advantage
- Diversify into new growth businesses
- Expand into new markets
- Apply R&D skills in new areas
- Enter new related business
- Vertically integrate forward or backward
- Enlarge corporate portfolio
- Overcome barriers to entry
- Reduce rivalry among competitors
- Make profitable new acquisitions
- Apply brand name capital in new areas
- Seek fast growth market

TABLE 1-4. SWOT Threats — Environmental

- Attacks on core business
- Increase in competition
- Change in consumer tastes
- Fall in barriers to entry
- Rise in new or substitute service
- Increase in industry rivalry
- New forms of industry competition
- Potential for takeover
- Existence of corporate raiders
- Increase in regional competition
- Changes in demographics
- Changes in economics
- Downturn in economy
- Rising labor costs
- Slower market growth

As we dive deeper into this honest assessment of your practice, there are some additional key areas to review:

Organizational structure
- Do we have the right legal arrangement to meet professional and taxation issues?
- Should we join another group, sell, or take the lead in expansion?
- Does our current organizational structure work? Is it divisional or departmental or location specific? Are controls, communication models, and decision-making levels defined, and do they work well?
- Do we have a process in place for annual review?

Location
- Is the current office location the best?
- Are we meeting the needs of the patients that we serve?
- Should we expand or contract our locations to optimize our efficiency and/or to best serve our patients?

Credentials
- Is our paperwork up to date – licensure, DEA?
- Do we have a structure in place to ensure nothing falls through the cracks and all required credentials are in place, regularly reviewed and updated?
- Do we have a system in place to effectively add a new provider?
- Do we have a process in place for annual review?

Accounting and reporting
- Does the existing financial accounting and reporting system work?
- Do we have checks and balances in place?
- Do we get timely information to allow for decision making and effective communication to all owners?
- Is staffing adequate, well trained, and effective in communication?
- Does the budget development, reporting, and updating process work?
- Do we know, understand, and control costs?
- Is the revenue cycle optimal?
- Do we have a process in place for annual review?

Fee schedule
- Is the current fee schedule appropriate for Medicare and all payer contracts?
- Do we manage private payment options appropriately?
- Do we review our schedule, at least once annually?

Coding
- Do we have the necessary resources available to answer any questions?
- Do we review coding decisions and documentation regularly? How?
- Do we track denials or other issues around coding?
- Do we have a compliance system in place to address outliers?
- Do we have a process in place for annual review?

Software
- Do we have the right EMR and PMS systems; how effective is the interface?
- Do we have appropriate maintenance agreements?
- Do we have a cybersecurity system in place?
- Do we receive adequate training and support from our vendor(s)?
- Is there anything else required to interface with practice areas?
- Do we have a process in place for annual review?

Communication
- Do we have the right telephone system?
- Does the answering service work?
- Do we have adequate cell phone use, policy for use, and security in place?
- Does the internet work?
- Do patients have access to internet in reception area? Does that requirement affect staff use and do we have a policy in place on access?
- How effective is the patient portal?
- Do we have a process in place for annual review?

Equipment and supplies
- Do we have the right operational equipment?
- Do we have the right ancillary equipment?
- Do we have maintenance agreements?
- How do we control inventory?
- Do we have checks and balances for controls on ordering and inventory?
- Do we have a process in place for annual review?

Marketing
- How effective is our marketing program?
- Do we use social media effectively?
- Do we have an annual budget in place?
- Are we serving the right population?
- Do we have adequate reporting and analysis to ensure optimal market penetration?
- Do we have a process in place for annual review?

Operations
- Do our processes work?
- Is scheduling, handling of new patients, tracking follow up visits effective?
- What is our cycle time per provider and location?
- What is the third new patient available slot per provider?
- Does our interdepartmental transfer of patients and data work?
- Do we have a process in place for annual review?

Insurance
- Do we have adequate insurance to cover disaster, business loss, fire, cybersecurity, and the like?
- Do we have the right agent(s)?
- Do we have a process in place for annual review?

Human resources
- What is our staffing ratio this year compared to last year?
- Do we have the right metrics to measure staffing levels?
- Do we have an effective staff training program?
- Do we have an appropriate benefit package? Is it well documented in the employee handbook?
- Do we have effective recruitment, selection, on boarding, and retention?
- Do we have an effective discipline program?
- Do we pay adequately?
- Do we have a process in place for annual review?

Compliance/Quality
- Does our compliance program work?
- Does it cover all necessary areas to meet federal and state regulations?
- Do we adequately monitor compliance with all internal policies and procedures?
- Do we emphasize quality?
- Do we have evidence based treatment plans in place?
- Do we monitor and manage internal and patient safety programs?
- Do we have a process in place for annual review?

Let's compare this honest assessment of the practice to something more familiar. The training of a physician includes not only looking at the patient's condition, but to look at the symptoms and then deeper to the etiology. We can apply the same approach when assessing a practice. When looking at the practice, we must consider:

Practice condition
- Review of assessment checklist (at end of Chapter 1)
- What are the key performance indicators, KPI? (Financial statement, turnover, patient visits)
- What are the patient satisfaction scores?

Symptoms
- Too busy
- Not enough provider time
- Low inventory
- Things are never is the right place
- Crisis hire pattern

Etiology
- Unclear mission
- Confused or multiple cultures
- Poor talent, staff hiring, and retention

This list is intended to start your thought process on how effective and efficient your practice currently works. It is not a complete list. The gaps should give you a roadmap to improvement. You should use the following chapters as a reference to enhance your understanding and to look for helpful hints on how to improve in the areas noted by your gap analysis.

ASSESSMENT CHECKLIST

	Who's Responsible	Status
Organizational and Physician Issues		
Review legal firm, accounting firm		
Evaluate organizational options		
Structure buy/sell agreement, if group practice		
Review employment agreements		
Physician compensation model and employment agreements, if group practice		
Review organization structure for accountability and decision making		
Identify relationships with others - friends and competitors		
Location Analysis and Space Planning		
Conduct location analysis		
Determine space requirements		
Select location		
Re-negotiate lease terms if necessary and applicable		
Review office layout		
Evaluate space plans		
Review room by room supplies and fixed asset list		
Review signage		
Credentialing and Privileging Issues		
Determine present participation in plans & hospital privileges by provider - create matrix for annual review		
Review managed-care contracts, appropriateness, payment amounts and terms		
Review membership in state/county medical association/specialty societies		
Review state medical license		
Review federal narcotic license		
Review state narcotic license		
Competency of staff and systems for maintenance		

Financial Planning, Accounting and Billing Issues		
Annual budget		
Review loan financing requirements		
Review banking services needed and satisfaction/dissatisfaction with current bank		
Review merchant credit card account		
Review accounting system and related training		
Review practice internal controls		
Review petty cash policy		
Review practice management software system		.
Check clearinghouse for timeliness and reporting		
Review collection agency performance and internal referral process		
Review internal controls procedures		
Review revenue cycle - KPI status, reporting, and policies		
Review compliance with contract terms and regulations		
Fees and Coding		
Review usage of evaluation & management codes		
Review office charge ticket/procedure		
Review hospital charge process		
Review practice fee schedule		
Conduct CPT and ICD-10 training - determine need		
Review audit policy and results for proper coding, determine compliance and penalty plan		
Computer/Software Selection		
Review what's new and what might benefit patients and operations		
Define hardware & software requirements (e.g. PPM, EMR, imaging)		
Review software service agreements		
Do we have enough support - personnel and contracts?		
Review system adequacy for today and future		
Review computer training schedule and implementation timeline		
Communications – Digital, Internal		
Define hardware needs and update plan		

Determine lines/features needed		
Review internet, broadband capabilities, policies		
Review answering service, policies on text, messaging		
Review cybersecurity program		
Capital Equipment Planning		
Review needs - clerical and clinical		
Review furniture & equipment budget		
Determine acquisition schedule for new items		
Review examination room equipment		
Review other clinical equipment needs		
Review of instruments/smaller items - need and handling		
Review maintenance agreements		
Marketing Issues		
Review practice marketing plan and ROI		
Look at logo and overall image		
Review list of referring doctors and trends		
Review brochure and website/patient portal		
Review letterhead/business card design		
Are meetings necessary with referring sources?		
Effectiveness of staff engagement program		
Forms & Supplies		
Review new patient information forms		
Review patient portal - update and utilization		
Review process to obtain information from payers, e.g. NCD, LCD		
Check for current CPT and ICD-10 book		
Review inventory and ordering process of medical supplies		
Review pharmaceutical representatives policy and adherence		
Operational Issues		
Review ALL office policy and procedures		
Effectiveness of scheduling schema per provider and office		
Review month end procedures for timeliness and completeness		
Review daily/monthly financial reporting		
Review appointment scheduling guidelines and change procedures		

Review billing and accounts receivable follow-up guidelines		
Review financial policies		
Review all collection policies		
Review EMR processes		
Update patient cycle time per provider		
Review/revise periodic audit schedule		
Review accounts payable procedures		
Review financial statement and all monthly reporting dashboards		
Insurance Needs		
Evaluate insurance needs - disaster, recovery, cybersecurity, auto		
Review insurance agent's performance		
Review employee and personal coverage - disability, health, dental		
Review key person coverage		
Review business owner's policy		
Review employee fidelity bond coverage and related matters		
Human Resources		
Review staff positions ratio per provider or other benchmarks		
Review job descriptions and duties, revision plan if appropriate		
Assess current organizational chart		
Review wage and salary schedule		
Review personnel policy manual (PPM)		
Review employee benefit package		
Review hiring process - recruitment, selection and onboarding		
Review discipline and termination processes		
Review employee personnel files - accuracy, compliance and security		
Review employee training programs and budget		
Review payroll services		
Compliance and Quality		
Does the culture support compliance and quality initiatives and procedures?		
Review outside reference lab		
Ensure OSHA compliance		
Ensure CLIA compliance if applicable		

Ensure HIPAA compliance		
Ensure ADA compliance		
Ensure Stark compliance, if applicable		
Ensure compliance with MACRA		
Ensure compliance with care plan models practice wide		
Review for physician coverage		
Review reception room periodicals, internet, cleanliness		
Set up system for annual review of above		

Chapter 2

Patients: Customer Engagement and Patient-Focused Care

"The patient is our business," is a rather profound statement for many of those involved in providing care. Let's refer to an internet search of the definition of patient. According to dictionary.com, consider these definitions:

- Noun: "A person who is under medical care or treatment" or Archaic – "A sufferer or victim"
- Adjective: Bearing provocation, annoyance, misfortune, delay, hardship, pain, etc. with fortitude and calm and without complaint, anger or the like."[1]

These definitions help us understand what it means to be a patient in today's medical environment. There is so much pressure to see as many patients as possible, do as much possible for each patient, make sure the right steps are taken for the patient and family, and meet patient's needs, while at the same time trying to survive in the business of medicine.

Unfortunately, even I have been a "victim of the system" on many occasions. Here are some experiences I have had when seeking treatment as a patient:

- I had a retinal detachment issue. I called my ophthalmologist office on Wednesday when I couldn't see through my right eye. I was told they could not see me until Friday at 1:15! By that time, I had found a retinal surgeon and already had surgery. I talked with the doctor afterwards, who said I should have called her directly, as she is always available. Although I was thankful for her words, no one gave me her number or any way to contact her.
- I had an experience in-patient: I experienced a range of weak service including wrong size compression stocking, rusty IV pole, poor meals, a call system not working, and room temperature issues. I was also awakened at 3:30 AM for blood draw and again at 4:00 AM to have vital signs taken, indicating no real strategy or process.
- I needed to see cardiologist for surgical clearance. I couldn't get in until after the date of surgery per central scheduling staff, so I went to see another. When I discussed this issue after the procedure, I was told I should have called directly, and they would have worked me into the schedule. Yet there was no prior indication on how to do this.

- I had an orthopedic surgeon post-surgical visit. I scheduled this visit for 8:45 AM. When I talked with the surgeon at discharge, I was told he could only see me at 8:00 AM same day. I asked if I should change the appointment. His answer was no and that he " . . . always runs late anyhow!"

Although not my personal experiences, I have also heard many accounts of other patient issues. Two additional examples are:

- A patient that had sudden hearing loss and needed MRI. There was a 15-minute treatment slot, so the patient was given a go ahead. The patient's history indicated she had stents. Therefore, a special MRI was needed. The appointment was set up, and the patient arrived at the imaging center. At that time, she was told she would need to go to another center.
- A patient with small cancerous lesion in lung. The oncologist requests stereotactic radiation but realizes the patient could experience a cracked rib. The oncologist suggests that another alternative is cyro therapy, which works well with problems in the lung. This option was not discussed initially. Was this because of time limits, or interest in radiation center options?

I could go on, but how many of these types of instances have you heard of or experienced yourself? My key question is: have we gotten so big and so uncaring that we have forgotten about the basic patient needs?

Back to my first sentence of this chapter: the patient is our business. A business defines customers as "a person who purchases goods or services from another . . . *informal* . . . a person one has to deal with."[2] Our patients are purchasing services (through a third party) and is the one whom we deal with directly.

From the perspective of the practice, it is interesting to consider where the patient fits and what impacts the patient interaction with the health care system. Figure 2-1 reflects the many items that impact the patient interactions with the system and raises questions for the practice. What are you doing to address all these influences, while maintaining a focus on the center of your business model - the patient?

PATIENT-FOCUSED CARE

Many pundits have indicated that the healthcare system is physician-centric. Efforts have been underway to change this with the evolution of the PCMH, the ACO and variations created by health care systems. Instead of disputing the physician-centric question and identifying the best model, I suggest there is no best model. Instead the concept or philosophy that should be part and parcel of each physician practice should be patient-focused care, PFC.

The American Academy of Pediatrics proposed the development of a medical home in 1992 "which refers to delivery of advanced primary care with the goal of addressing and

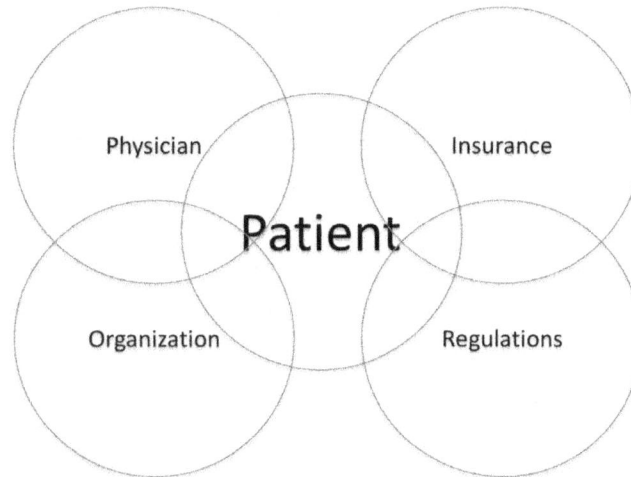

FIGURE 2-1. Influences that Impact the Patient

integrating high quality health promotion, acute care and chronic condition management in a planned, coordinated, and family-centered manner."[3] Several reasons have been cited for why this has been difficult to develop, the main reason revolving around reimbursement. However, today the concept has taken on new meaning with several initiatives.

The Institute of Medicine in its landmark report *Crossing the Quality Chasm* emphasized the development of "patient-centeredness" as a key aim in US healthcare delivery. These developments lead to the establishment of the Triple Aim supported by the Institute for Healthcare Improvement, which emphasizes access, quality and cost control in all policies developed and implemented. This has become the mantra for many of the discussions around the ACA and the many attempts to repeal and/or revise. Here again, we wish to bring this to the level of the individual practice and consider if you practice patient-focused care daily?

The Picker Institute working with The Commonwealth Fund in 2007 published a paper addressing "What Does it Take?" to achieve implementation of the patient-centered medical home in inpatient and outpatient settings. There were six core elements noted:

1. Education and shared knowledge
2. Involvement of family and friends
3. Collaboration and team management
4. Sensitivity to nonmedical and spiritual dimensions of care
5. Respect for patients needs and preferences
6. Free flow and accessibility of information[4]

These elements should make up your practice plan for addressing the patient-focused aspect of providing care. We have expanded this list in the checklist for Patient-Focused Care at the end of this chapter.

It is interesting that this list encompasses not only the direct medical needs and understanding but expands to include the family and non-direct medical needs of the patient. It suggests treating the whole patient and not simply the symptoms or disease state. This broadens the responsibility, but also leads to improved outcomes and patient satisfaction.

A point that is missing from the list is the medical outcome for the patient. What is a satisfactory outcome for the patient?

Health Outcomes are a change in the health status of an individual, group or population which is attributable to a planned intervention or series of interventions, regardless of whether such an intervention was intended to change health status.

Such a definition emphasizes the outcome of planned interventions (as opposed, for example, to incidental exposure to risk), and that outcomes may be for individuals, groups or whole populations . . . Health outcomes will normally be assessed using health indicators.

As a non-clinician, I cannot comment on the medical aspect. But I simply offer the fact that the health outcome of the treatment approach and plan is critical, in addition to how the experience in the care process was managed.

CMS does identify seven key outcome measures offering some guidelines for consideration in the approach to individual patient care:[5]

1. Mortality – life expectancy
2. Readmissions
3. Safety in care provided – in office and in hospital
4. Patient experience
5. Effectiveness of care – compliance with evidence based, best practices and overall outcomes on key treatment plans
6. Timeliness of care – access to provider
7. Efficient use of imaging

How and what do we do to provide those services in a satisfactory manner? Let's look at the mechanism available to gauge if we are satisfying a patient.

SATISFACTION AND SURVEYS

When considering the popular concept of satisfaction surveys remember that it is the patient's experience that starts the process. The experience leads to the satisfaction score. The experience starts well before the patient visits the office. It starts with the phone call or on-line experience of setting up the appointment. Similarly, the process ends not necessarily with the check out, but with the conclusion of the final payment for the services provided. The satisfaction does not always lead to a quality experience. It is also the health outcome that is important. A positive experience may lead to high satisfaction, but negative outcomes and vice versa.

The survey strategy must be well thought out. From a strategic perspective there are several points to keep in mind when considering a satisfaction survey approach:

1. What is the key measurement for satisfaction? Factors for consideration include the quality of care, the physician interaction, the staff, the call to schedule, and wait time in the office.

2. What attributes should be in focus? Some factors include ambience of the waiting area, engagement of staff, time with physician, and so on.

3. What benefits should the patient expect from the experience, or rather, what is your hypothesis on what the actual survey outcome will be?

4. How will the results be tabulated? Will the results be informational or actionable? Note that the more actionable the results, the more directed the improvement effort will be.

5. What follow up will occur from the results gathered? What will the team do with the results? Will there be publication of the results, as well as what has been done with them?

Basically, surveys are designed to obtain information from a customer about the product or service they have purchased. These can be conducted in person, via snail mail, email, drop box link, or via telephone calls. The approach is up to you. The goal should be to achieve feedback - negative or positive. Many surveys include a Likert scale from one to five, excellent to poor, or some variation of those terms.

It is not just important to obtain the ranking. It is necessary to find out what is behind the ranking choice made by the one who responds to the survey. If you have hundreds of responses that list your service as a 5, what does that tell you? What if they are all 1s? Did you meet the customer's expectations? Did you do it well? What part of the customer service process was excellent, and what did not meet their expectations?

How do you know what the patient's expectations were? Were they upset with the wait time? Did they expect more personal contact, or more time with the provider? Did they expect to be treated with respect, and maybe greeted personally? Or did they expect to have their medical needs met? We often hear that every patient is different. making it impossible to meet their expectations. Thus, all we can do is our best.

If two patients present in the same hour with the same symptoms, do you treat them the same? The question really evolves around two different issues – does one have more complexity, e.g., co-morbidities, while the other has no other factors? Expand this to include if one has time pressures and the other one does not. The former is an 84-year old female who uses the office visit to see people. The latter is a 30-year old attorney who needs to get back to work. One requires significant clinical experience, the other requires an efficient process. This breaks down the different needs and outcomes. What system issues are similar, and which are different? Do you do well in each case? We'll address efficiency issues in a later chapter. For now, consider, the complexities around understanding patient satisfaction with the visit.

A practice will be surveyed by the Federal Government program (CG-CAHPS for practices and HCAHPS for hospitals) with results available through various CMS and DHHS websites. Each payer surveys patients about their experiences as well. There are private organizations such as Press-Ganey and SullivanLuallin which offer survey instruments and comparison options for your practice with others in their data base.

But you can also develop your own survey instrument. When doing so use caution on the questions and refer to your strategic perspective. This ensures that the right questions are asked, and actionable information is obtained.

Typically, a Likert scale of 1 – 5 is recommended, as more options will complicate the response. Use of excellent, good, poor or words of this nature may also be used. Some sample questions:

- Overall how would you rate the quality of service you received today?
- How often have you visited the office in the past year or past six months?
- How would you rate our concern for your privacy and transparency?
- How would you rate the professionalism of the staff?

The big one:

- Based on today's visit would you recommend our practice (doctor) to a family member or friend?

You can leave space for comments related to each question. Personally, I believe that the shorter the survey the better. Long surveys tend to be less accurate and more "tiresome" for the patient to complete. Long surveys both via snail mail and email can get frustrating to complete and in a recent case I experienced, the email survey featured many redundant/related questions. When I got frustrated, I simply quit the survey! It is possible to adjust your questions regularly (quarterly) to focus on one or two key areas of concern. The targeted number of responses per survey is open ended and you should check the recommendations on the web for targeted percentage returns. A minimum of 30 responses is desired.

Also check the web for social media action from resources like Facebook, Yelp, and Health Grades. It is not advisable to respond directly to comments made, but to use this as a supplemental source of information to assist your "repair" plans.

Hospitals and medical practices make mistakes in their efforts to monitor and obtain information via satisfaction surveys. These include not having a clear focus on the standards and expectations, not communicating with employees on the plan and their role, not holding management and staff accountable for the program, being too aggressive toward staff when there is no improvement in the care delivered, poor communication, and unclear focus and understanding of the priorities and who is responsible for what.[6] Obviously, these key mistakes are not universal, but warrant consideration as the strategic plan is developed.

Studies like the 2012 study published in the *Archives of Internal Medicine*, have noted that to satisfy patients, physicians have ordered unnecessary procedures and driven up costs of healthcare. This involves more hospital admissions and increased drug costs.[7]

Another word of caution: any survey data gathered may be admissible in court. So, make sure you have a system in place to deal with recommendations and comments for improvements. A team of staff members should review the data with a structured follow-up and documentation program in place. Whether or not you publicize results, or actions taken from results, is up to you. The more transparent the practice and the more proactive the practice is in responding, the more beneficial this process is to the practice.

GENERATIONAL AND CULTURAL DIFFERENCES

It would not be uncommon for a practice to care for all four generations and/or patients from different cultures on the same day. This requires an understanding of several factors to ensure effective communication and successful outcomes from the treatment plan.

A quick look at generations are noted in the following table:[8]

TABLE 2-1. Generational Characteristics

	Traditional	Baby Boomers	Generation X	Millennials
Core values	Respect for authority Conformers Discipline	Optimism Involvement	Skepticism Fun Informality	Realism Confidence Extreme fun Social
Family	Traditional Nuclear	Disintegrating	Latch-key kids	Merged families
Education	A dream	A birthright	A way to get there	An incredible expense
Communication Media	Rotary phones One-to-one	Touch tone Call me anytime	Cell phones email	Internet Smart phones Text
Dealing with money	Put it away Pay cash	Buy now, pay later	Cautious, conservative, Save, save	Earn to spend

Each different patient generation comes with some built in perspectives as noted in the Table 2-1. This generalization is not to put everyone in the same bucket, but to caution the reader to consider these perspectives when addressing the patient and their needs.

In addition to the generational issues, the diverse nature of the population in the United States suggest that an awareness of cultural differences found throughout the globe also need to be considered. We talk a lot about culture in this book, mostly looking at the culture of the practice itself. Here we focus on the patient - their background, and the related values. When considering the "customer" as a patient, there are several dichotomies which are worth reviewing.[9] See Table 2-2.

TABLE 2-2. Cultural Characteristics

Dimension	Defined	How to deal	Area
Neutral vs.	No emotion, poker face	Control your emotions, understand the customer	Japan British
Emotional	Show their emotions	Use expressions, don't be overwhelmed with emotional gesture	Netherlands, Mexico, Italy, Spain
Universalist vs.	Expect to be treated like everyone else	Treat with clear set of rules, objective	US, Canada Australia, Germany
Particularist	Expect more privilege built on personal relationships	Personal relationships, grant special privileges	China, Russia, Indonesia
High context vs.	Messages implied not stated	Pay attention to hidden, subtle messages, beware of double meanings	Japan, France, Russia
Low context	Explicit, simple, clear, straightforward	Take customer at face value, be simple and precise	US, Canada, Netherlands, Germany
Individualist vs.	All are individuals, more important than group	Individual stands out, respect personal decision making	US, Netherlands
Community	What people think of you is important, social hierarchy	Focus on relationship, patient needs to fit in	Germany, China, France, Japan
Achievement vs.	Self-value based upon what you have done	Respect status, focus on data	US, Austria, Israel, UK, Switzerland
Ascription	Where from, age	Show respect for age, power, position, mention titles	India, China, Indonesia

Deductive vs.	Theories, deeper concepts presented	Explain theory and deeper meaning	Italy, France, Spain, Russia
Inductive	Focus on practical such as fact or opinion	Be practical, avoid theoretical arguments	US, Canada, UK, Netherlands
High Power Distance vs.	Ask to speak to the manager, act authoritatively	Respect their position, don't expect empowered employee can solve problem	China, Japan Russia, Saudi Arabia
Low Power Distance	Don't value authority	Don't mention their position, allow others to solve problems	Denmark, Sweden, Australia
Negative Feedback vs.	Direct	Don't be shocked, be clear, negative doesn't mean loss of patient	Netherlands, Germany, Israel
Positive Feedback	Subtle and polite	Be perceptive to what sounds like a suggestion, be gentle	China, Saudi Arabia, Mexico
Linear scheduling vs.	Future is planned, tight deadline, perfect execution	Be precise and explicit in the treatment plan	Germany, Mexico, Japan
Flexible	Fluid future, plan is an intention and subject to change	Be flexible and recognize response to treatment plan may not be perfect	India, Saudi Arabia, China

This is a lot to take in, but when you consider your patient experience and the patient's background/culture, these dimensions and their contrasts make sense.

PATIENT ENGAGEMENT

What is engagement when we consider an individual? Patient engagement is fostered and measured by staff as well as the provider. Marcus Buckingham and Curt Coffman in *First Break All the Rules* spell out specific choices when it comes to developing or maintaining a relationship with another individual:

- What is expected and what is received?
- What do I get as a patient by coming to this practice?
- Do I belong here? Are these people my friends?
- How can I get better by seeking care in this practice?

Communication between staff, provider, and the patient is key in addressing each of these questions. Each question could be asked differently, from the perspective of each staff member. They should be asking what they can give, are they friendly, can they do better in meeting the needs of the patient, and do they meet the patient's expectations. Staff members that are engaged can fix, influence, and enhance the engagement simply by being more attentive to the needs of the patient.

Communication with the patient can be perceived based upon body language, tone of voice, or the words used. First impressions are formed almost immediately, within seven seconds. Successfully achieving engagement is centered on how well the staff is trained in this area. Practicing communication methods, awareness of what is being said and how it is being said, will help ensure compliance with treatment plans. Going beyond this, reflective listening where staff repeats their understanding of what the patient stated will help achieve engagement.

Hopefully the mission of the practice is well-defined and communicated to staff. That mission should include quality of care and an engaged approach to the patient. With this mission, and corresponding values, the patient will be received and treated well - meeting their expectations.

Patients will bring a preconceived notion on what will happen, as noted above, based upon generation and/or culture. Some other factors to consider are the patient's transportation (how difficult is it for the patient to get to the office, do they have internet for telemedicine?), their finances (will they fill the prescription and follow the instructions, or cut pills in half to get twice the time frame?), and if the staff educate the patient (if so, do you offer the type of education approach that will work for each patient?) As noted throughout, a single standard approach may seem efficient, but may not wholly work.

Some patients may be dismissive, yell, cry, be scared, or have other emotions that surface when told about their diagnosis or treatment plan. The staff must recognize these reactions and be trained to respond appropriately and in a timely manner.

Let's look at all the above in the context of today's healthcare world which goes well beyond the individual. We have value-based care, evidence-based care, and population management. The payer world, including Medicare, have focused on data gathering via processes that occur or don't occur in the office. Health Effectiveness and Data Information Set, HEDIS, payer Star ratings, and standardized core quality measures are all designed to measure both processes and outcomes. More focus has occurred on processes.

A process is a check and balance idea where data is submitted when a criterion is met, or something is done, e.g., HbA1C quarterly for diabetic patients. There is no real guarantee of an outcome based upon this simple measure. An outcome measures the patient's condition and health status, typically over a long period of time.

Clayton M. Christensen, in his book *The Innovator's Prescription* offers a very interesting perspective when we look at the patient and why they come to the office. The basic idea is that a patient comes to the office seeking care, and a cause of action is to seek what you can do. This is the trigger and is the cause for what *needs to be done*. The outcome or goal is *adherence to the need* to have provided the service. The goal of every encounter should be beyond getting a good patient satisfaction score. It is to create a state of well-being for every patient who seeks services, acute, chronic or wellness based.

We also must consider what the practice is doing regarding the needs of the community. This includes understanding and assisting the community in areas of obesity, opioid management, transportation, mental health, and anything else pertinent to the practice's community. The key point here is that while engaging the patient, the understanding of the age and culture mix of the community is a responsibility of the practice, as well. This can be enhanced with a solid working relationship with the payers and how both parties work to measure success through processes and outcomes.

PATIENT PARTICIPATION IN DECISION MAKING

Expanding on the concept of engagement lies the question of the role of the patient in decision making in their own care. There are several benefits for patient participation in decision making including, but not limited to:

- Increased satisfaction and trust
- Improved quality of life
- Better understanding of requirements for managing their care
- Improved compliance with the care plan
- Increase acceptance of their responsibility in the receipt of care

There are different approaches that the physician can take in dealing with patient participation. The physician can be autocratic, insisting that there be no participation, and that the way determined by the physician is the only way to be considered. The opposite extreme is that the patient makes the decision and the physician accepts and acts accordingly. The middle of the road is when there is a mutual decision made between the physician and the patient. There are multiple factors that will help direct the process. Such factors include the degree of listening of all parties involved, extent of knowledge and assurance of the accuracy of the diagnostic process, the patient's quality of life expectations, patient's family, and the evidence available related to the options available for the treatment plan. There is no one best way for the physician to approach the patient's situation. Each circumstance is different. Experience and the perceptions of the physician will help lead to the best option. It is possible that a physician will use the two extremes and the middle of the road approach all within the same week. The key is that the physician be aware that today's patient has more information, is more proactive, and expects to be more involved than many of the older patients who may be in their care.

POPULATION HEALTH

One of the concepts in this book is that healthcare is changing and that a major focus is on the concept of population health. In the Introduction we talked about the value-based approach and the evolution to population health. The three components that are significant in management of the population are chronic patient needs, the wellness of the general population, and individualized care. Chronic care is expensive, involves several providers or care strategies, the need to coordinate care, and may evolve to various payment models, such as suggested by Christensen. The wellness concept moves from the current "sick care, fee-for-service model" to one focusing on keeping the patient well. This encourages not only regular checkups but encourages changes in lifestyle including nutrition and exercise and stress reduction. Individualized care returns to the current model, but in many ways is limited by the "15-minute" visit slot in the provider's schedule.

The Patient-Centered Primary Care Collaborative, PCPCC, has developed seven shared principles of primary care. We think these should be applied to all specialties considering the move to population health. These seven principles are:

1. Person and family centered – focus on the whole person, mutuality of the care team involvement including the patient and family.
2. Continuous – enduring relationships to ensure communication, perspective and proper context throughout all stages of life including end-of-life care.
3. Comprehensive and equitable – addressing and awareness of the whole person, social determinants, and customizing the care to the patient.
4. Team-based and collaborative – all work toward a common goal. Team members are trained in their skills but also trained to work together for the good of the patient.
5. Coordinated and integrated – involving not only the primary care provider but all disciplines necessary for the care of the patient. Coordinating through information exchanges and effective integration of all systems for efficient and effective communication.
6. Accessible – the vertical nature of facilities, from hospitals to surgical centers, and the horizontal nature of other facilities, such as the physician office, urgent care, retail clinic, home health, and telemedicine are all options for the patient to have access. The key is to ensure that the patient knows, and understands, the options available.
7. High value – effective and efficient use of resources to control costs.

This set of principles provides a great tone for moving into an effective delivery model for all providers.

BEHAVIORAL HEALTH

A special area of need that continues to surface is behavioral health. From school shootings, to the opioid crisis, to the long-known need to provide mental health care to individuals continues to highlight that this area is not well managed. Why?

The ACA and previous efforts such as the 1996 Mental Health Parity Act and the subsequent Mental Health Parity and Addiction Equity Act of 2008 have suggested that patient's behavioral health needs are not being met and that financing options are available. These have led to improved payment for services and recognition of various models for care delivery, the main points are to recognize that mental health is an issue, that there are ways to address patient needs, and that not only will health outcomes improve, but there will be significant cost savings.[10]

- "Many behavioral and physical disorders are co-occurring, especially depression and chronic medical conditions."
- "There are often better mental health outcomes when physical problems are managed."
- "Addressing psychological aspects of problems presented in primary care often results in lower overall health costs."
- "Offering behavioral health services in nontraditional settings encourages participation by people wanting to avoid the stigma surrounding mental health treatment."
- "Seven of the ten leading causes of death (heart disease, cancer, stroke, chronic lower respiratory disease, accidents, diabetes, and suicide) have psychological and/or behavioral component."
- "70% of all health care visits are generated by psychological factors."
- "An estimated 75% of patients with depression present physical complaints as the reason they seek health care."
- "When family physicians worked collaboratively with mental health professionals to treat persons on short-term mental health disability leave, their patients returned to work at higher rates than those treated by physicians alone. The average cost savings to employers was $503 per patient."
- "In addition, some of the most effective adjunctive treatments for problems like chronic pain, irritable bowel syndrome, and hypertension involve evidence-based psychosocial interventions – those that aren't medications, devices, or medical procedures."[11]

The key message here is that mental health is an issue impacting roughly 25% of all US citizens and that the needs of these patients, at least from a mental health perspective, largely go untreated.

The provider's awareness of the behavioral needs of patients is the first step. But what are the best ways to address these needs in the 15-minute visit, to seek options for care? Perhaps integrating a behavioral health question or two into the intake or basic questions during the initial physical interview will help. There are models that can work. Any practice can refer out or collaborate with a behavioral health specialist. The second option is to co-locate, meaning share space in the office with a behavioral health specialist. The third option is to hire qualified personnel as part of the physical medical side of the practice. We will review these models in greater detail in the business chapter.

REFERENCES

1. Dictionary.com. Accessed December 1. 2018.
2. Dictionary.com. Accessed December 1, 2018.
3. American Academy of Pediatrics, Medical Home. https://www.aap.org/en-us/professional-resources/practice-transformation/medicalhome/Pages/home.aspx. Accessed December 1, 2018.
4. Shaller D. Patient Centered Care: What Does It Take?, The Commonwealth Fund; October 2007; https://www.commonwealthfund.org/publications/fund-reports/2007/oct/patient-centered-care-what-does-it-take. Accessed December 1, 2018.
5. Tinker A. The Top 7 Outcome Measurements and Measurement Essentials. Health Catalyst; https://www.healthcatalyst.com/knowledge-center/insights/category/analytic-in-healthcare/. Accessed December 1. 2018.
6. Gamble M. 6 Mistakes Hospitals Make in Patient Satisfaction Efforts. *Becker Hospital Review*; https://www.beckershospitalreview.com/hospital-management-administration/6-mistakes-hospitals-make-in-patient-satisfaction-efforts.html. Accessed December 1, 2018
7. UC Davis Health. Patient Satisfaction Linked to Higher Health-Care Expense and Mortality. UC Davis Health News; February 13, 2012; https://www.ucdmc.ucdavis.edu/publish/news/newsroom/6223. Accessed December 1, 2018.
8. Hammill G. Mixing and Managing Four Generations of Employees. *FDU Magazine*; Winter 2005. https://www.fdu.edu/newspubs/magazine/05ws/generations.htm. Accessed December 1. 2018.
9. Understanding Cultural Diversity in Customer Service. Userlike; September 21, 2016; https://www.userlike.com/en/blog/cultural-diversity-customer-service. Accessed December 1. 2018.
10. http://www.ibhpartners.org/. Accessed December 1, 2018.
11. Corso K, Hunter C, Dahl O, Kallenberg G, Manson L. *Integrating Behavioral Health into the Medical Home*. Phoenix, MD: Greenbranch Publishing, 2016.

CHECKLIST FOR PATIENT-FOCUSED CARE

Education and shared knowledge • In reception area • In exam room • Brochures • Digital		
Involvement of family and friends • Welcome to visits • Meeting space • Outreach		
Collaboration and team management • Who is responsible • Frequency of discussion in meetings • New program developed • Search for new resources		
Sensitivity to nonmedical and spiritual dimensions of care • Integration of support		
Respect for patients needs and preferences		
Free flow and accessibility of information		

Use role plays to help staff understand and become more engaged:

- You are at home alone in the afternoon and having major pain. This is an emergency. What do you do?
- You need to get to your doctor's appointment. You don't have a car and you are feeling too weak to take public transportation. How do you get there?
- You are meeting a new doctor for the first time alone, without your family. The doctors asks you to tell him/her about yourself, your chronic illness, your medical history, and the current medications you are taking. Let's switch roles. What does the doctor ask? Now, how do you respond?
- You are having some symptoms that could be related to your chronic illness, although you are not sure. What do you do next?
- You just met with your doctor. You are unclear about something that was discussed during your visit and this is upsetting you. What should you do?

Source: http://www.bostonleah.org/PDF/transition_roleplays.pdf

Chapter 3

The People Factor: Recruiting and Keeping Good Staff Members

When you look at a medical practice's financial statement, one of the first things you notice is the cost of payroll and associated benefits. This can easily exceed 25% when measured against total revenue (varies by specialty). One of the bigger costs of managing staff is the cost of turnover. Many studies find that this ranges from 70% to 200% of the individual annual salary. Additionally, many surveys have identified a level of engagement, or rather disengagement, of employees in their job, which results in poor productivity. The point here is that effective management of individuals in the medical practice must be a key focal point.

To set the tone, it is necessary to consider the culture within which the staff functions. Surprisingly, the Department of Health and Human Services has a definition that is applicable here. Culture is defined as "Integrated patterns of human behavior that include the language, thoughts, communications, actions, customs, beliefs, values and institutions of racial, ethnic, religious and social groups."[1] Each point made in this definition has an impact on the daily lives of each, and every, employee. The culture is established by the practice leadership through words and deeds. Culture is a powerful driving force in the success of a practice.

GENERATIONAL AND GLOBAL WORK FORCE

As noted in the previous chapter, it is not uncommon for a practice to have four different generations in the practice environment. Beyond the generational differences, there are gender differences. There is also a distinct possibility of a racial mix. Within the possibility of a racial mix, there may also be a mix of nationalities. These breakdowns of our differences are not intended to create a tension, but rather to challenge you to consider how you manage and maximize a diverse team to achieve the real goal of providing, and improving, patient care.

Table 3-1 offers insight into the generational issues that are faced.[2] The categories are based upon birth years: traditional (1945 or earlier), baby boomers (1946 – 1964), Generation X (1965 – 1980), and millennial (1981 – 1997). There are other ranges, but these are the most typical when searching for breakdowns and definitions. A key point to understand when reviewing the table below is that this is a broad overview of characteristics. The people within these generations will not always automatically fit into these categories. Not everyone born into their category will act the same way.

TABLE 3-1. Broad Characteristics of Generations

	Traditional	**Baby Boomers**	**Generation X**	**Millennial**
Work ethic and values	Hard work Respect authority Sacrifice Duty before fun Adhere to rules	Workaholics Work efficiently Crusading causes Personal fulfillment Desire quality Question authority	Eliminate the task Self-reliance Want structure and direction Skeptical	What's next Multitasking Tenacity Entrepreneurial tolerant Goal oriented
Work is . . .	An obligation	An exciting adventure	A difficult challenge A contract	A means to an end Fulfillment
Leadership style	Directive Command and control	Consensual Collegial	Everyone is the same Challenge others Ask why	Evolving
Interactive style	Individual	Team player Loves to have meetings	Entrepreneur	Participative
Communication	Formal Memo	In person	Direct Immediate	E-mail. Text Voice mail
Feedback and rewards	No news is good news Satisfaction in a job well done	Don't appreciate it Money Title recognition	Sorry to interrupt but how am I doing? Freedom is the best reward	Whenever I want it, at the push of a button Meaningful work
Messages that motivate	Your experience is respected	You are valued You are needed	Do it your way Forget the rules	You will work with other bright, creative people
Work and family life	Ne'er the twain shall meet	No balance Work to live	Balance	Balance

Continuing to dive deeper into the breakdown of our differences, our national culture is one with several nationalities and religions, each with their own specific characteristics.

You can take the extreme approach and decide that you do not want to have different generations or ethnicities within your practice. Or, you can accept the fact that these differences are unavoidable, and instead, benefit from different ideas and approaches to the practice mission. Staff members will live in their culture outside of work. They then bring those beliefs to the work place, which directly impacts the internal culture. Consider these points that impact management decisions and actions:[3]

- Communicating: explicit versus implicit
- Evaluating: direct negative feedback versus indirect negative feedback
- Leading: egalitarian versus hierarchical
- Deciding: consensual versus top-down
- Disagreeing: confrontation versus avoidance
- Persuading: holistic versus specific
- Scheduling: organized time versus flexible time
- Trusting: task versus relationship

With this information in mind, the need then becomes to develop intercultural sensitivity to the staff.

Dr. Milton Bennett created a "Developmental Model of Intercultural Sensitivity" (DMIS) in which he cited six stages.[4] Consider each of these to determine where you are as an individual, but also where your overall practice stands.

- Denial – no differences
- Defense/reversal – recognition of difference but stick to your own, or vice versa and attempt to bend the other way
- Minimization – yes, there are differences, but they don't impact us
- Acceptance – understand and value differences
- Adaptation – temporarily beginning the process of integration
- Integration – fully established approach and policies recognizing the differences

After recognition of where you are, it is necessary to develop a programmatic approach to achieve integration. A formal training program for management, and eventually evolving to the staff, is a key step. This can involve external sources for discussion, open exchanges between staff members, role plays, and much more. In this program discussion, there should also be a focus on communication between employees. Concise messaging, avoiding slang and certain expressions, listening, and respect for cultural and religious differences are vital when communicating with employees. As with generational differences in communication models, be aware of verbal, written, and non-verbal ways of sending and receiving messages.

To use a recent example to further strengthen the importance of developing a programmatic approach, let's refer to the disclosures of sexual harassment incidents and the evolution of the #metoo movement. In the practice environment, the predominant support structure is female, while historically the dominant physician player has been male. There have been many instances, both open and silenced, of harassment. While not citing any here, it is important that respect for each other, both as individuals and the role necessary to provide patient care, is kept in mind. A clear policy, open and non-threatening pathway to discussion, and annual reviews and training on this issue must be part of any practice.

RECRUITMENT

Let's talk about recruitment. In many cases, there is an immediate need to fill an open position, which may result in a "crisis" hire. Picture this: on a Thursday afternoon, the receptionist resigns and walks out. On Friday, the first person that walks in the door to interview is hired and starts work on Monday. They are greeted, shown where the phone is, told the name of the practice, and is asked to begin helping with the responsibilities. By noon, they leave. Even more, an established patient is overheard making a comment that there is another new person at the front desk. Does this sound familiar? Does this solve a problem, or create more?

To avoid situations like this, it is important to do the same deep dive into recruitment at your practice. What is your process for hiring? Do you utilize employees to refer (preferably engaged employees), use one of many internet search options, post notices at the local coffee shop, or another way to source applicants? What is the cost of this search?

Who screens the applicants? Do you have a human resources department, and if so, what is their role? Who coordinates the interview process?

Here are some hints for this process that will, most likely, always help:
- The manager makes the hiring decision.
- The applicant is screened for "personality" or fit, and not so much for skills (unless licensure or certification is required). It is easier to train and enhance skills than it is to change a personality.
- Delay - do not crisis hire since the real goal is long term stability in the position, rather than finding a just anyone to occupy the position.

In the interview process, consider what you are really looking for. Obviously, licensure and certification are critical for certain positions. Beyond that, I always think of the personality of the individual. As mentioned, this is based on the understanding that you can train skills but will struggle with changing the personality. But note - many organizations have used personality tests to screen individuals. I am not a proponent of these since this may color the judgement of the interviewer.

Instead, structure the interview in a specific way. Make the setting comfortable so the candidate will be relaxed. Don't sit behind the desk (implies a power position), but, instead, have a face-to-face comfortable setting with no barrier. Ask the basic questions about background, etc. to ensure that what is noted on the resume or application form is consistent with what is being said. Get the candidate to talk about themselves.

Ask the candidate to describe circumstances they have experienced. When interviewing for a receptionist, ask how they handled an angry or emotionally distraught situation. Or, how they handled a happy mom to be. Get them to share how they reacted and how they phrased their approach in a variety of different situations. This will help you determine if their personality and approach will be a good fit with the rest of the team.

ONBOARDING

Once the candidate has accepted the job, make sure to recognize the applicant, now employee, as an asset or investment. You must not overlook, or skimp, on the orientation and training effort. Make certain that the first one to six weeks of employment includes:

- Introduction to practice by someone in leadership
- Review of benefits
- Identify the individual mentor for each new employee
- Introduction and welcome to the department; socialize with others
- Work environment
- Work schedule and tasks associated with the position
- Technology – access to, how to use, and policies
- Encourage input by asking questions like: this is how we do it, do you have experience or suggestions on doing it better?
- Sequence over a time period; this is not a one-day thing

BEYOND ONBOARDING

Many of the younger generation, the Millennials, as identified earlier, will make up at least 50% of the workforce by 2020. These individuals are looking for education, training, and the opportunity for growth in their jobs. Therefore, you must question the investment and approach your practice is taking to meet this growing demand. Very often, the educational budget goes to the professionals who travel to conferences. Very little is directed toward growth of the support staff, and new employees. This can be addressed in several ways:

- Webinars – many "free" or inexpensive options are available. Some are hosted by vendors of products currently used in your practice or are offered as value add or marketing to switch to their product. Some offered for a fee by reputable organizations. This can also reach several staff members at the same time. The excuse that you can't take several staff members out of the flow is real, but efforts should be made to work around this with cross training or shifts in the schedule for that time.

- Hiring training staff – there are many highly skilled individuals who are eager to train and have skill sets related to teaching. Not all practices can afford this option, but training consortiums, working with hospitals and federally qualified health centers, where resources may be more readily available, is a viable option.
- Mentoring programs – identify key employees who do a great job and recognize them by asking them to assume the role of mentors for the new employee, or the recently promoted employee. These individuals should be trained in the role, and a well-defined job description, with checklists to follow in the process, should be developed. Reward both the mentor and mentee when completed.
- Coaching programs – this is different than mentoring in that this is the responsibility of management to coach the employees. You don't see the baseball coach at shortstop while the game is being played, but you do see them talking to the player in between innings. This is a broader, more collective approach. A coaching role should be always in the forefront of the mind of every manager.

PERFORMANCE REVIEW

Traditionally, performance reviews occur after 90-days of employment and annually thereafter. This is the opportunity for the manager to meet with the employee to review their performance, and to set the tone for the expectations into the following year.

The most common approach is bi-directional, or a self and manager evaluation. Each party reviews the annual performance with the manager considering the input from the staff member. Typically, the annual increase is then based upon the final decision made by the manager, or in some cases the CEO, President, or the entire board.

Some management consultants note that these evaluations do not provide any improvement in performance and are a waste of time. Today's generational issues indicate that the old way may work for baby boomers but may not work with the younger generations.

It is more important to frequently intervene with the employee, rather than wait for the annual review. In order to reinforce behavior expected, it is more effective to coach the employee at the time a situation occurs. This includes praise to reinforce positive behavior, especially when done in front of others to gain maximum benefit, as well as addressing behavior that is not appropriate or acceptable privately. Both positive and negative incidents are teachable moments and should be noted in the employee's record.

CROSS TRAIN AND PROMOTE

Staff members can do more than one job. There is a constant need, due to illness or volume fluctuations, to have staff trained to do more than what is identified in their job descriptions.

Why can't the receptionist be taught to obtain vital signs, or the medical assistant trained to greet and register a patient? Obviously, there are restrictions where licensure tasks are involved, but even then, licensed staff can be taught to assist in other key aspects of providing care.

Another good example is to cross train billing staff to do the front desk duties, and vice versa. This is not only good for flexibility, but also for awareness of how important it is to capture the right data, collect at the time of visit, understand insurance.

Keep in mind that promotion from within is an aspiration of many staff members. While attempting to control turnover of staff and reduce that cost, creating an environment where opportunities to move on may help your practice to retain a good asset. This can be accomplished and enhanced by developing a learning organization.

LICENSURE, CERTIFICATION AND WORKING TO YOUR LEVEL OF KNOWLEDGE AND SKILL

There continues to be discussion about the limited number of available physicians to serve increasing demand. Supply and demand, and burnout, are factors in this issue. More to the point, the practice needs to continually recognize the knowledge and skills of staff members. For example, as the nurse practitioner and physician assistant roles continue to evolve, licensing processes evolve as well. It is key to recognize the talent of these individuals, and to utilize them appropriately. In many cases they can handle their own patient load, helping offset the increasing demand of service.

Other specialty trained providers such, as pharmacists, can assist in the more complex world of dispensing and drug interactions. An often-overlooked area is behavior specialists. With nearly 25% of the US population suffering from mental health issues, this is a major area of undersupply.

ENGAGEMENT

Stephen J. Swenson, M.D., medical director for leadership and organization development at the Mayo Clinic in Rochester, Minnesota, has identified six ways to bring joy and seek engagement in their organization:[5]
1. Encourage leaders to support and engage with employees.
2. Include staff in decisions and leadership seeks out their opinions.
3. Build a sense of camaraderie.
4. Identify and address the major drivers of stress and burnout.
5. Find ways for staff members to support one another.
6. Promote both physical and metal resilience among employees.

A concept that was identified in 1990, by William A. Kahn, is the idea of employee engagement.[6] This is more than asking if the employee is satisfied with their work and their employer. This digs deeper into the idea of the employee's emotional connection and willingness to commit to the work at hand.

There are several definitions of employee engagement, here is a good one from Forbes: " . . . the emotional commitment the employee has to the organization and its goals."[7]

The Forbes article suggests that engaged employees will lead to higher services, higher customer satisfaction, increased sales, higher level of profits, and higher shareholder returns. I would always argue that the best outcome is focused on customer satisfaction, since satisfied customers lead to higher profits.

The Gallup organization has surveyed employees in virtually every industry since the mid-90's. The outcome has been similar:
- 18% fully disengaged
- 52% disengaged
- 30% engaged

The Gallup survey mentioned above contains 12 questions.[8] These have been included here and are not intended to be used to survey your staff, but rather to give you a sense of the questions asked in a Gallup survey. If you desire, please contact Gallup to conduct a survey for your practice.

Gallup survey questions:
1. Do I know what is expected of me at work?
2. Do I have the materials and equipment I need to do my work correctly?
3. At work, do I can do what I do best every day?
4. In the last seven days, have I received praise for doing good work?
5. Does my supervisor, or someone at work, seem to care about me?
6. Is there someone at work who encourages my development?
7. At work, do my opinions seem to count?
8. Does the mission of my company make me feel my job is important?
9. Are my co-workers committed to doing quality work?
10. Do I have a best friend at work?
11. In the last six months, has someone at work talked to me about my progress?
12. This last year, have I had opportunities at work to learn and grow?

There are some truly amazing results, such as that any organization could have 70% of its employees not committed to the organization, but instead just simply going through the motions of accomplishing tasks daily. Additional data suggests that 69% of all disengaged employees would leave the practice for a 5% increase in wages. And a 20% increase will lure those fully engaged.[9] When reviewing these statistics, the important question to ask is why? Is there something that can be done to invert that ranking in your practice?

Saba Software produced a 2017 State of Employee Engagement survey based on results from over 1,800 responses from the US and the UK.[10]

They found 58% of employees were not asked for feedback very often, sometimes only infrequently throughout the year. Another 58% result shows that employees think their concerns won't be addressed quickly, while 51% of their concerns will be dismissed outright. Another major finding that directly impacts the medical practice was that 57% of women were comfortable giving feedback, versus 64% for men.

It is essential to take an honest look at yourself and your practice with the results mentioned above in mind. The Saba survey offered specific survey differences between what "HR leaders" (translate this to all managers) felt about certain matters compared to employees (Table 3-2).

TABLE 3-2. Staff Engagement Survey

	HR	Employee
Training and Development		
Training and development are accessible and effective	80%	67%
Training provided is effective in developing and advancing careers	80%	65%
Social Learning and Collaboration		
Organizations provide effective forums for collaboration	72%	51%
Performance Management		
Performance review process is helpful	75%	46%

Effective engagement management programs include several key points:

- Senior leadership must communicate a clear vision and purpose – make sure all staff members know what is key, and what is important to the culture of the practice. Make sure to highlight whether it is more important to make money, provide quality care, provide a safe environment, provide a learning environment for employees to grow and prosper, or anything else that makes up the vision and purpose of the practice.
- Train, but don't make it a "new program." When introducing a training initiative, it is important to acknowledge that many new processes will stick for a few weeks, but then may be forgotten. As mentioned above, multi-cultural and multi-generational issues are present, but don't forget they're present with patients as well. Finding fun ways to share thoughts and ideas, noting that nothing is "stupid." Facilitating an open environment in all educational programs will lead to success.

- Communicate – it is important to communicate who you are, what your key performance standards are, and what is expected – and to review these regularly. More importantly, it is important to encourage staff to get involved. Staff should be encouraged to solicit ideas for improvement, enhance engagement with patients, listen and respond to what is being said or written. Giving information, and respecting information that is coming back, will go a long way in continued engagement of staff.
- Empower staff – give them more authority and control over their work. Who better to improve than those that do the job? A simple way of both improving communication and empowering staff is to question *why* they do the task, or *why they do it in a certain way*. One strategy is to repeat the why question up to five times to get to the root cause of the issue and/or a solution.
- Hold staff accountable and recognize when successful – if an idea has surfaced, or the staff has done an excellent job in engaging patients, recognize that effort. In today's value-based payment world, show the employee that they contribute and that the practice values their contribution.
- Be available – management is busy trying to manage many tasks and interruptions. A concept that may work is to have an open-door policy, but not an open clock. This means setting aside some time to catch up on other things and minimize interruptions. Focusing on them will encourage further engagement.
- Trust – open communication, respect, consistency, and responsiveness will lead to a level of trust with staff members.
- Senior leaders – don't just say it, live it!

We purposely have not labeled, or listed, the physician in the above discussion. Even though the implication is they are part of senior leadership, it is as important, if not more, for the physician to be engaged with patients and employees.

PHYSICIAN/PROVIDER/CLINICIAN

In order to respect all definitions of the above classifications, all will be referred to as physician for this section. Obviously, the key staff member in the organization is the physician. Even though others influence the patient and the care system, the weight of the physician portion of the encounter is paramount. With issues facing not only medical care, but quality metrics, updating the EHR, reimbursement, population health management, etc., simply stopping and talking with the patient seems like a bother. Yet engagement with the patient - looking them in the eye, listening to their issues, explaining the care plan - will result in compliance and a highly satisfied patient visit.

As we discuss engagement, we must also discuss malpractice. Risk management points include these:

1. Communicate – the two parts of communication can be broken down to the sender and receiver. You have a message, but you also must listen to what is being said. Explaining the care plan, supplementing it with educational materials in paper or online, having staff support and discuss the plan, ensuring that all questions are answered and documenting what was said and done, are all important in avoidance of a malpractice claim.

2. Practice reflective listening – ask the patient to repeat what you just said to make sure they understand the expectations as a result of the visit, or procedure.

3. Be nice – respect the patient and family members. Don't rush.

4. Prepare for the visit – look at the chart, see the picture, remember something from a previous visit like the name of a pet, or a hobby or career.

5. Medical and social awareness while relating to the patient, is a winner.

6. Remember to follow up with the patient – examples include having the staff call after the procedure to see how things are going, and letting the patient know the results of a test. Make sure to be thorough with the follow up, which could mean confirming they get the message, even for normal test results.

7. Think like a patient – what would you like to know?

8. Be consistent.

9. Stay up to date with the latest – be prepared for something coming from an internet search.

10. Obtain consents for services, if necessary - train staff and check with your malpractice carrier to ensure proper forms and procedures are in place.

11. Don't be afraid to ask for help from an associate!

Now if we switch gears to look at engagement, many of these same concepts will meet that objective. A 2015 study by PLOS ONE identified a list of physician communication skills most desired by patients:[11]

- Empathy
- Careful listening
- An open mind
- Friendliness
- Compassion
- A genuine interest in the patient
- Attentiveness
- Willingness to ask questions and initiate conversations
- Investing time and effort to educate patients and make sure they understand the illness

Taking both lists in consideration as you look at individual patients within the context of population health, we see a tendency to consider the whole person and their wellbeing. A key point to realize is that each individual visit can, and will, have an impact on the population management approach.

Patients today, regardless of age, are interested in understanding more and more about their disease. Differing from years past, they can now obtain information on the internet. If they come with a certain expectation based on their research, you need to be able to successfully listen, and then direct them to a more appropriate understanding of what the best plan is for them. Involving family and/or care givers in this process is essential, as well.

A 2016 Health Reform Monitoring Survey provided some interesting insights related to physician communication with patients. They found that most non-elderly patients had a high trust factor, 9-10 on a 10-point Likert scale, with the median 7-8. However, as noted above, when related to culture needs, one-third of the minority racial/ethnic patients were below the median, as compared to one-fifth of the white, non-Hispanic patients.

The survey asked about potentially sensitive issues including "health and health care challenges," concerns about cost, and events that may cause stress or worry in daily lives. 90.2 percent were comfortable discussing at least one sensitive issue. Note that the highest responses were related to health, and the lowest were related to "life challenges" and costs. Again, there was a gap between white, non-Hispanic and minority/ethnic patients' perspectives.[12]

There also was a gap in provider-initiated discussions, with only 61.2 percent of patients reported provider initiation of sensitive issues, and 53.2 percent on life challenges. This points to the question of time available, and focus of the physician on the issues, while in the exam room. We will discuss this more in Chapter 6.

A key aspect of any relationship is the level of trust that is established. It takes a few seconds, in any relationship, to begin forming the level of trust that will exist between the two parties. As we investigate the individual relationship, we find that the focus has changed. Earlier, e.g., in the 1970's, physicians were more like parents, by telling patients what the plan was and how it would work. Today, with access to so much information, the relationship between the physician and the patient is more of a partnership. This partnership is further tempered by the fact that insurance is in the middle.

Many patients are new to insurance as part of the ACA. Recent studies have been conducted to help identify what insurance is elected, why it is chosen, and what is expected from insurance by patients. Few, if any, conclusions have been identified. Yet one key question is raised regarding the measurement of the physician/ patient relationship as a result of these studies.

The key to all the above is to determine whether the patient has been compliant with the treatment plan. Current efforts relate to patient education (brochures, internet), reminders to take medications, and even financial incentives through insurance. However, as we consider population health, as well as the individual patient health, there are social factors such as overall literacy, access to care, and overall distrust in the system, that impact the outcome.[13]

At this point, the best that can be done is for an internal effort to not only develop care plans, but to identify key aspects of compliance over time. This requires physician-to physician-discussion, and an honest assessment of the infrastructure available to track the necessary data points. This may seem like a lot to do, but when you consider that there are care models available and that the goal is to achieve quality of life outcomes, it is the responsibility of the practice to take necessary steps now. This will put the practice ahead of the curve. It will also work on behalf of the practice in negotiations with payers through improved data and partnering.

PHYSICIAN BURNOUT

A lot has been written lately about the pressures, subsequent stress, and burnout faced by physicians/clinicians today. The long-term stress reaction by an individual developed by emotional wear and tear, loss of personal contact, and decreased sense of personal accomplishment lead to burnout. This leads to questions about treatment plans, patient safety, and patient access to care as outcomes from the daily stress faced by physicians.

The Agency for Healthcare Research and Quality, AHRQ, has sponsored major projects on the working conditions of all healthcare professionals. They have found, as well as others, major causes for burnout:[14]

- Time pressure
- Chaotic environment
- Low control of the pace of the daily practice
- Electronic Health Record, EHR
- Balance all with family

They add to this an unfavorable work culture, which all lead to dissatisfaction with the practice of medicine. This reaction to the many external pressures, faced by physicians, have led to closing practices, leaving their individual practice, and even an increase in suicide.

AHRQ suggests there are some interventions, which are promising to prevent or reduce physician burnout. These include:

- Flexible work schedules
- More time
- Work life balance
- EHR entry assistance

One of the goals of this book is to help the physician reduce overall stress. This cannot be done by making the day 26 hours. Rather, it can be done by making the time spent more efficient. Using the tool TAKT Time, which measures time available to meet the demand placed upon it, we find that if a physician works an eight-hour day and sees 25 patients, the time available for each patient is 19.2 minutes. Reduce that time to six hours in the clinic, and the time available for each patient is 14 minutes. Ask yourself, is it even possible to see 25 patients? When you consider the primary care specialties and sub-specialists with limited clinic time and the demand placed upon them by the system, reducing the number of patients is not a viable option.

Therefore, it is wise to consider what is being done to support the physician. Sure, flexible schedules can help, as noted by AHRQ but, again, that does not offer the balance of the demand placed upon each provider. As you continue to read this book, you will find assistance in how to be more efficient, and how staff can work more closely with each provider to support. Instead of two hours of pajama time doing records every night, maybe reassigning staff to eliminate duties from the provider is a possible option.

Work life balance can be done by simply agreeing with associates that one evening per week will mean taking nothing home, instead of just being removed from the call schedule. Another option would be to agree that after 8 PM every night, when not on call, there will be no more electronics. This is helpful when recommending another suggested cure - getting some better sleep!

The topic of physician health should be regularly discussed at physician meetings. Techniques, hints, re-working individual work load, standardizing support systems, reflecting on the earlier discussion on how to manage staff, focusing on becoming a learning and more efficient organization and the like will go a long way toward reducing individual stress.

SUCCESSION PLAN

From burnout we turn to a succession plan. This may be a touchy subject to many senior physicians and long-term executives. But it is critical to have a solid succession plan in place. This is not just for the "C suite" or President. This should be for everyone in the organization and should incorporate a philosophy you develop for staff to replace yourself and any other position. This should not be viewed as a threat, as it is key to long term success, and will ultimately resemble that of a legacy. Not to be morbid, but what would happen to the organization if something happened to you this evening, and you no longer could work? What has been done to prepare your business for that occurrence?

Sure, the business would continue, but how smooth, how successful, and at what cost depends on the type of succession plan you have in place. It is essential that leadership develop a solid succession plan, and that this is part of the annual review and update process. You need to review what has been done, and what needs to be done to develop, communicate, and ensure success.

Here's a simple list of things to consider for each position, and as a model for your succession plan:[15]

- Create or revise a job description – your own and those who may follow. Include in YOUR job description the concept of mentoring and/or coaching.
- Train – develop a learning organization culture and don't be afraid to include in the annual budget funds for external training programs and networking.
- Create milestones – a point in time to review to determine the readiness of the individual to take over.
- Focus on the future, not just today – discussions, awareness of the many changes in the population health movement, behavioral health needs, value-based, capital expenditures, and so much more. These topics should be reviewed regularly with your successor.
- Don't clone yourself – let them be themselves but hone their skills to meet the needs of the future.
- Share with others – let your team know what is expected, who is involved, and why things are moving forward. This may create jealousy or competition but being transparent is better than surprising the team later.
- Constantly communicate – keep your successor and team well informed on the plans of the business and, since retirement is an option, your personal plans.

The key point here is to plan, prepare, and to not be afraid of developing and embracing the future. It will come with, or without, a succession plan. The implications of future events will be better if you prepared.

TEAM BUILDING AND WORK

Purposely left to the end of this chapter are the ideas of team work, leadership, and management. Why? The horizon leading to future success in population health and value-based models requires all to work together under effective and efficient leadership.

Let's tackle the team first, which can be defined as "A group of people with a full set of complementary skills required to compete a task, job, or project."[16] It is no longer possible in this highly complex world for one person to know and do everything required to achieve positive outcomes in every circumstance. Hence, working with, and through others, is necessary.

The effective team goes back to points made earlier about recruiting, selection, and retention of key individuals with knowledge, skills, and the right attitude fit. Missing in the above definition is the need to work together to complete the project. Thus, attitude is an essential aspect of a successful organization.

The team process typically follows four stages:
- **Forming** – selection of the right members who will assist in accomplishing the goals of the team. The number required varies based on the extent of need for knowledge and skills to accomplish the goal. Typically, no less than three, and no more than seven.

You may ask for assistance from others to supply information, provide insights, or guide as the sequence proceeds.

- **Storming** – no one gets along or there is one who does not fit. The team leader role is to identify and smooth over any "personal" disagreements. Disagreements themselves when focused on the topic at hand are acceptable, it's the attitude, or inner workings, of the team at this stage that must be addressed immediately and effectively.
- **Norming** – when the team moves past the previous two stages and begins its work toward accomplishment of the goal.
- **Performing** – a smooth running machine, all members are syncing together, and the process is proceeding to successful fulfillment of its goal.

A fifth stage is often considered when using teams for projects that are not permanent in nature. This stage is adjourning, meaning that there is an end. It is at this point that an evaluation of the team process, what worked and what didn't, are noted. This learning moment is critical for the leader, as well as the team members who will, assumedly, be involved in other teams in the future.

When recognizing the second stage, storming, it is important to note that there are many personalities that surface in the team process and may surface at any time. There is the dominant personality, who is typically controlling and attempting to win their point of view. There is the constant talker, who has a comment or opinion on everything. These types must be controlled, allowed to make their "factual" points, but not dominate. There can be the shy one, who has knowledge and skills, but is afraid to speak up. Typically, this type of personality has a lot to contribute. Encouraging involvement in a non-threatening way will help them feel comfortable speaking up.

As a team leader it is important to recognize the stages of teamwork, and to set the tone. This typically means having agendas, rules, and minutes for each meeting that occurs. Start the meeting on time, e.g., 1:29 vs. 1:30, and end on time, e.g. allowing 59 minutes for the meeting. Set time limits for each major point on the agenda, e.g., 10 minutes. Establish that speaking limits are 1 – 2 minutes per member, per topic. Each member must say something of substance at each meeting, not necessarily on each point on the agenda. Keep minutes. Circulate the agenda prior to the meeting, and the minutes after to keep everyone focused on what is happening. Meetings can be a significant waste of time if not managed properly.

LEADERSHIP AND MANAGEMENT

A quick definition of leadership is doing the right thing, while management is doing things right. Another of my favorite definitions of management is working with, and through, people to achieve desired results. There is a subtle difference in leadership and management that must be recognized. It is possible to be both a good leader and manager, but it

TABLE 3-3. Levels of Leadership

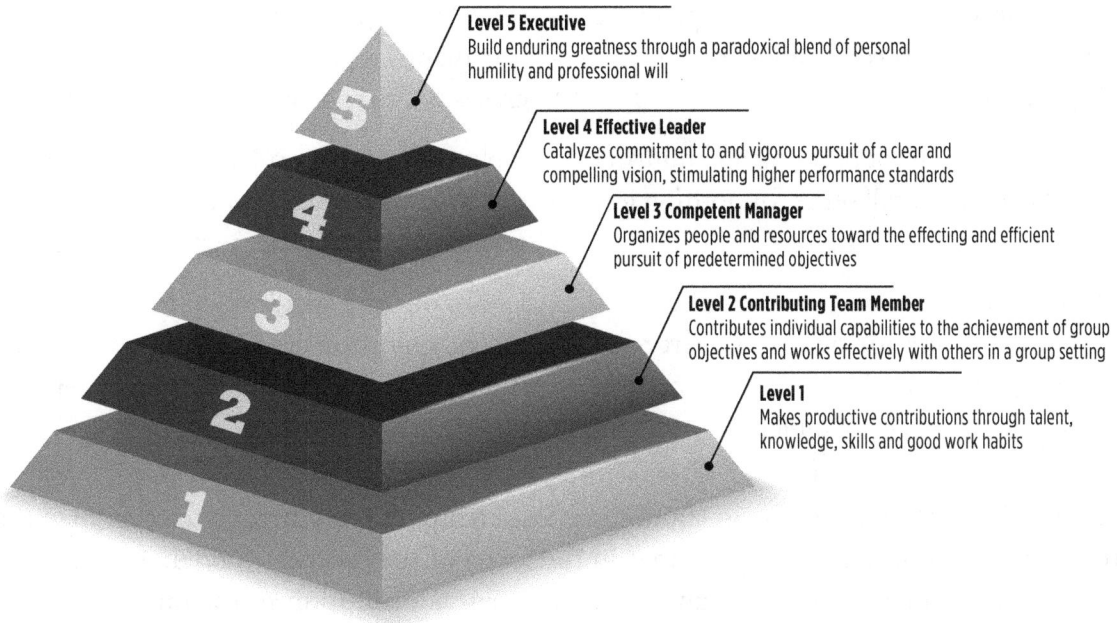

Level 5 Executive
Build enduring greatness through a paradoxical blend of personal humility and professional will

Level 4 Effective Leader
Catalyzes commitment to and vigorous pursuit of a clear and compelling vision, stimulating higher performance standards

Level 3 Competent Manager
Organizes people and resources toward the effecting and efficient pursuit of predetermined objectives

Level 2 Contributing Team Member
Contributes individual capabilities to the achievement of group objectives and works effectively with others in a group setting

Level 1
Makes productive contributions through talent, knowledge, skills and good work habits

is also possible to be one, and not the other. Recognizing your role, skills, and knowledge is essential. Jim Collins in his book *Good to Great* helps clarify these points in his pyramid related to the idea of Level 5 leadership in Table 3-3.[17]

This display is in a pyramid structure with Level 5 being at the TOP of the pyramid.

While reflecting on this section, and the previous section on team work, review each level noted on the pyramid. All levels are essential, and it is possible that many of you have progressed through each level to achieve Level 5! The Level 5 leader, according to Collins, focuses on the organization and channels "their ego needs away from themselves and into the larger goal of building a great company." This returns to the key point that the attitude, personality, or chemistry created by the leader will set the tone, and consequently, filter through the organization.

Collins identifies two sides of Level 5 Leadership:[17]

Professional Will	Personal Humility
Creates superb results, a clear catalyst in the transition from good to great	Demonstrates a compelling modesty, shunning public adulation; never boastful

Demonstrates an unwavering resolve to do whatever must be done to produce the best long-term results, no matter how difficult	Acts with quiet, calm determination; relies principally on inspired standards, not inspiring standards, not inspiring charisma, to motivate
Set the standard of building an enduring great company; will settle for nothing less	Channels ambition into the company, not the self; sets up successors for even greater success in the next generation
Looks in the mirror, not out the window, to apportion responsibility for poor results, never blaming other people, external factors, or bad luck	Looks out the window, not in the mirror, to apportion credit for the success of the company – to other people, external factors, and good luck

Not to be critical of physician training or leadership, the key here is to recognize that others are important. This suggests that in the arena of the business model, working with and through people, recognizing and accepting their contribution to the outcomes of the overall patient care picture, leads to success.

REFERENCES

1. US Department of Health and Human Services, Office of Minority Health, 2013. What is Cultural Competency? https://minorityhealth.hhs.gov/omh/content.aspx?ID=2804. Accessed December 1, 2018.
2. Hammill G. Mixing and Managing Four Generations of Employees. *FDU Magazine*; Winter 2005. https://www.fdu.edu/newspubs/magazine/05ws/generations.htm
3. Meyer E. Cross-Cultural Diversity Challenging Global Managers. March 11, 2013; https://www.shrm.org/resourcesandtools/hr-topics/global-hr/pages/cross-cultural-diversity-global-managers.aspx. Accessed December 1, 2018.
4. Bennett M. Developmental Model of Intercultural Sensitivity (DMIS); https://en.wikipedia.org/wiki/Bennett_scale. Accessed December 1, 2018.
5. Minemyer P. How WellStar Health System Improved Staff Engagement. September 14, 2017; https://www.fiercehealthcare.com/healthcare/how-wellstar-health-system-improved-staff-engagement? Accessed December 1, 2018.
6. Rheem D. William Kahn: Father of Employee Engagement. January 12, 2018. https://donrheem.com/william-kahn-father-of-employee-engagement/. Accessed December 1, 2018.
7. Krause K. What is Employee Engagement? *Forbes*, June 22, 2012. https://www.forbes.com/sites/kevinkruse/2012/06/22/employee-engagement-what-and-why/. Accessed December 1, 2018.
8. Feld C. Gallup's 12 Questions to Measure Employee Engagement; February 3, 2011; https://christopherfeld.wordpress.com/?s=gallup+survey+questions&x=0&y=0. Accessed December 1, 2018.
9. Dale Carnegie White Paper, Building a Culture of Engagement: The Importance of Senior Leadership. http://www.dalecarnegie.ca/wp-content/files/remote/Building_a_Culture-_The_Importance_of_Senior_Leadership.pdf. Accessed December 1, 2018.

10. SABA 2017 State of Employee Engagement Report. http://www1.saba.com/StateofEmployeeEngagement Report2017.html. Accessed December 1, 2018.

11. Rocque R. Leanza Y. A Systematic Review of Patients' Experiences in Communicating with Primary Care Physicians: Intercultural Encounters and a Balance between Vulnerability and Integrity, PLOS ONE, October 6, 2015. https://journals.plos.org/plosone/article?id=10.1371/journal.pone.0139577. Accessed December 1, 2018

12. Long S, Bart L, Hempstead K. Patient-Centered Care Starts with Patient-Provider Communication. *Health Affairs*. September 22, 2017; https://www.healthaffairs.org/do/10.1377/hblog20170922.062078/full/. Accessed December 1, 2018.

13. Blumenthal D, Yu-Isenberg K, Yee J, Jena A. Real-World Evidence Complements Randomized Controlled Trials in Clinical Decision Making. September 27, 2017. https://www.healthaffairs.org/do/10.1377/hblog20170927.062176/full/. Accessed December 1, 2018.

14. Agency for Healthcare Research and Quality, Physician Burnout; https://www.ahrq.gov/professionals/clinicians-providers/ahrq-works/burnout/index.html. Accessed December 1, 2018

15. Clark T. 8 Steps to Plan for Your Successor. Liquid Planner, August 13, 2013; https://www.liquidplanner.com/blog/8-steps-to-plan-for-your-successor/. Accessed December 1, 2018

16. http://www.businessdictionary.com/definition/team.html. Accessed December 1, 2018

17. Collins J. *Good to Great*. New York, NY, HarperCollins, 2001.

FOR THE EMPLOYEE: JOB DESCRIPTION QUESTIONNAIRE

Please complete the necessary information and answer all questions to enable us to serve the needs of the practice and provide you with the best guidelines possible. This information will be used to draft job descriptions. *If additional space is needed, please key # and use reverse side.*

Name: _____ Job Title: _____ Supervisor: _____

Date: _____ Full time: _____ P/T # Hrs wk: _____

1) List basic qualifications necessary for your position (education, training, basic skill set, etc.):

   _____

   _____

2) List personality traits essential for this position (i.e. determination, congenial, team player, attention to detail etc.):

   _____

   _____

3a) List the main *general responsibilities* of your position (give time parameters). Do not describe every task. Simply list the major job tasks you are responsible for:

Task Description	Est. time spent each task	
	daily	weekly
1.		
2.		
3.		
4.		
5.		
6.		
7.		
8.		

3b) If there are any tasks which you perform that you think would be better performed by another employee, what are they and why?

_____

_____

4) What tasks do you perform to assist another individual in the office? Estimate how much time is spent doing this daily?

_____

_____

5) Describe the physical demands/requirements in your position. For example if lifting is requirement, how much weight?

_____

_____

CALCULATE YOUR COST OF TURNOVER

Turnover Cost Model		Example	Your actual
1	Annual Salary	$31,200.00	
2	Benefit cost	$6,552.00	
	Total employee cost	$37,752.00	
	Hourly rate	$18.15	
3	Separation costs	$500.00	
4	Vacancy costs	$726.00	
5	Costs to hire	$3,000.00	
6	Intro to job	$2,904.00	
	Total replacement costs	$7,130.00	
	Percent for employee	22.9%	

Comments and what is used for example
1. $15.00 per hour/2080 hours paid
2. 21% of salary
3. Exit interview, administration costs, separation pay (if any)
4. Replacement costs, overtime, temporary staff
5. Advertising, employee referral fee, interviews, background, reference, bonus, moving expenses (if any)
6. Onboarding and other training days/staff

Original based on several examples found on internet search

GETTING TO KNOW YOU

Name	
Job title:	
Spouse's name	
Children's names and ages	
Hometown	
Hobbies	
Favorite (dream) vacation	
Best accomplishments • Family • Personal • Childhood • Work	
Favorite holiday	
Favorite food(s)	
Other comments	

- Copy and distribute to all team members before the meeting.
- During the first meeting, team up asking one person to interview another and vice versa
- Share the top three things learned about the employee

ONBOARDING AND WELCOMING THE NEW EMPLOYEE

Before the Employee's Start Date

Outcomes: *This is to prepare a welcoming work environment with informed colleagues and a fully-equipped work space. New employees feel "settled in" on their first day.*

Schedule and Job Duties
- Submit the Hire transaction
- Call employee:
  - Confirm start date, time, place, parking, dress code, etc.
  - Identify computer needs and requirements.
  - Provide name of their onboarding buddy.
  - Remind employee to complete tasks on the New Hire Activity
- Add regularly scheduled meetings (e.g. staff and department) to employee's calendar.
- Prepare employee's calendar for the first two weeks.
- Plan the employee's first assignment.

Socialization
- Email department/team/functional area of the new hire. Include start date, employee's role, and bio. Copy the new employee, if appropriate.
- Set up meetings with critical people for the employee's first few weeks.
- Arrange for lunch with the appropriate person(s) or buddy for the first day and during first week.
- Select the buddy.
- Meet with the buddy, and provide suggestions and tips.
- Arrange for an office tour.

Work Environment
- Put together welcome packet from the department and include: job description, welcome letter, contact names and phone lists, practice map, parking and transportation information, mission and values of the organization, information on your unit/school, etc.
- Clean the work area, and set up cube/office space with supplies.
- Order office or work area keys.
- Order business cards and name plate.
- Arrange for parking, if needed.
- Add employee to relevant email lists.

Technology Access and Related
- Order technology equipment (computer, printer, iPad) and software.

- Contact local IT to have the system set up in advance.
- Arrange for access to common drives.
- Arrange for phone installation.

Training/Development
- Arrange pertinent trainings required for the job.

First Day

Outcomes: *The employee feels welcomed and prepared to start working; begins to understand the position and performance expectations.*

Schedule, Job Duties, and Expectations
- Clarify the first week's schedule, and confirm required and recommended training.
- Provide an overview of the functional area – its purpose, organizational structure, and goals.
- Review job description, outline of duties, and expectations.
- Describe how employee's job fits in the department, and how the job and department contribute to the unit.
- Review hours of work. Explain policies and procedures for overtime, use of vacation and sick time, holidays, etc. Explain any flexible work policies or procedures.

Socialization
- Be available to greet the employee on the first day.
- Introduce employee to others in the workplace.
- Introduce employee to his/her buddy.
- Take employee out to lunch.

Work Environment
- Give employee key(s) and building access card.
- Escort employee to Human Resources to complete I-9 and obtain ID.
- Discuss transportation and parking or escort employee to transportation office to obtain parking sticker.
- Provide department or building-specific safety and emergency information.
- Take employee on a office tour.
- Explain how to get additional supplies.

Technology Access and Related
- Provide information on setting up voicemail and computer.

First Week

Outcomes: *New employee builds knowledge of internal processes and performance expectations; feels settled into the new work environment.*

Schedule, Job Duties, and Expectations

- Give employee his/her initial assignment. (Make it something small and doable.)
- Debrief with employee after he/she attends initial meetings, attends training, and begins work on initial assignment. Also touch base quickly each day.
- Provide additional contextual information about the department and organization to increase understanding of the purpose, value add to practice, goals, and initiatives.
- Explain the annual performance review and goal-setting process.
- Review the process related to the probationary period.

Socialization

- Arrange for a personal welcome from the unit leader.

Technology Access and Related

- Ensure employee has fully functioning computer and systems access and understands how to use them.

First Month

Outcomes: *Employee is cognizant of his/her performance relative to the position and expectations; continues to develop, learn about the organization, and build relationships.*

Schedule, Job Duties, and Expectations

- Schedule and conduct regularly occurring one-on-one meetings.
- Continue to provide timely, on-going, meaningful "everyday feedback."
- Elicit feedback from the employee and be available to answer questions.
- Explain the performance management process and compensation system.
- Discuss performance and professional development goals. Give employee an additional assignment.

Socialization

- Continue introducing employee to key people and bring him/her to relevant events.
- Meet with employee and buddy to review first weeks and answer questions.
- Arrange for employee to take office tour (if not already completed).

Training and Development

- Ensure employee has attended Human Resources New Employee Orientation.
- Ensure employee is signed up for necessary training.

First Three Months

Outcomes: *Employee is becoming fully aware of his/her role and responsibilities, beginning to work independently and produce meaningful work. He/she continues to feel acclimated to the environment, both functionally and socially.*

Schedule, Job Duties, and Expectations
- Continue having regularly occurring one-on-one meetings.
- Meet for informal three-month performance check-in.
- Continue giving employee assignments that are challenging yet doable.
- Create written performance goals and professional development goals.
- Discuss appropriate flexible work options.

Socialization
- Have employee "shadow" you at meetings to get exposure to others and learn more about the department and organization.
- Have a check-in with the employee and buddy.
- Take employee out to lunch, and have informal conversation about how things are going.

Training and Development
- Ensure employee attended a New Employee Orientation session. Request the employee provide feedback on the sessions and share as appropriate.
- Ask if needed training is completed.
- Provide information about continued learning opportunities.

First Six Months

Outcomes: *Employee has gained momentum in producing deliverables, has begun to take the lead on some initiatives, and has built some relationships with peers as go-to partners. Employee feels confident and is engaged in new role while continuing to learn.*

Schedule, Job Duties, and Expectations
- Conduct six-month performance review.
- Review progress on performance goals and professional development goals.

Socialization
- Create an opportunity for employee to attend or be involved in an activity outside of his/her work area.
- Meet with employee and buddy at the end of their structured buddy-relationship. Discuss how things went and what else would be helpful for the employee.

First Year [Between Six And Twelve Months]

Outcomes: *Employee is fully engaged in new role – applies skills and knowledge, makes sound decisions, contributes to team goals, understands how his/her assignments affect others in the organization, and develops effective working relationships. He/she has a strong understanding of the practice mission and culture. Employee continues to be engaged in his/her role and has gained greater confidence in position; begins to take on additional assignments and works with some level of autonomy.*

Schedule, Job Duties, and Expectations
- Celebrate successes and recognition of employee's contributions.
- Continue providing regular informal feedback; provide formal feedback during the annual review process.
- Have a conversation with employee about his/her experience at the practice to date:
  - Extent to which employee's expectations of role and the practice align with reality.
  - Extent employee's skills and knowledge are being utilized and ways to better utilize them; what's working, what they need more of, etc.
  - Begin discussing the year ahead.

Socialization
- Support and encourage employee participating on either a or cross-functional team.
- Solicit employee's feedback and suggestions on ways to improve the onboarding experience. Do this one-on-one or with a small group of new employees.

Training and Development
- Discuss employee's professional development goals and identify relevant learning opportunities.

Based on:
https://welcome.mit.edu/sites/default/files/documents/manager_onboarding_checklists.docx

Chapter 4

Partnering, Communication, and the Supply Chain

A BROAD DEFINITION OF PHYSICIAN ENGAGEMENT:

"Physician engagement is a strategy aimed at creating stable relationships between physicians and hospitals or health systems and is a critical success factor for navigating the delivery system transformation. An engaged physician correlates with enhanced patient care, lower costs, greater efficiency, and improved patient safety, as well as higher physician satisfaction and retention."[1]

In this chapter, the focus is on those external relationships, and their critical nature. As the definition notes, stable relationships are the key, but we expand this beyond hospitals and health systems to include payers, and suppliers of equipment and supplies. To effectively manage the practice, leadership must be involved with, or at least have a solid understanding of, each relationship to successfully follow the strategic plan.

RELATIONSHIPS

Every day we talk with countless individuals, including patients, staff members, other providers, and vendors. All these individuals are treated as our customers, and we continually relate to them through each interaction. The technical aspect of the world with internet, blogs, emails, social web sites, etc. take away some of the personal, face-to-face, time that existed in the past. However, there is still a relationship between the one who sends the message, and the one who receives the message.

These relationships, personal and technological, require effort to develop, maintain, and enhance. Several years ago, an article, by David Wilson, was published suggesting that there are keys factors in building relationships.[2] These key factors are expanded in the Table 4-1. These keys will ensure success in personal, as well as in business, relationships.

Social Bonds

Mutual Goals

Power/dependence

Structural Bonds

Communication   →   Trust   →   Commitment

Consistency   Compliance

Compare   Cooperation
Alternatives

Compassion

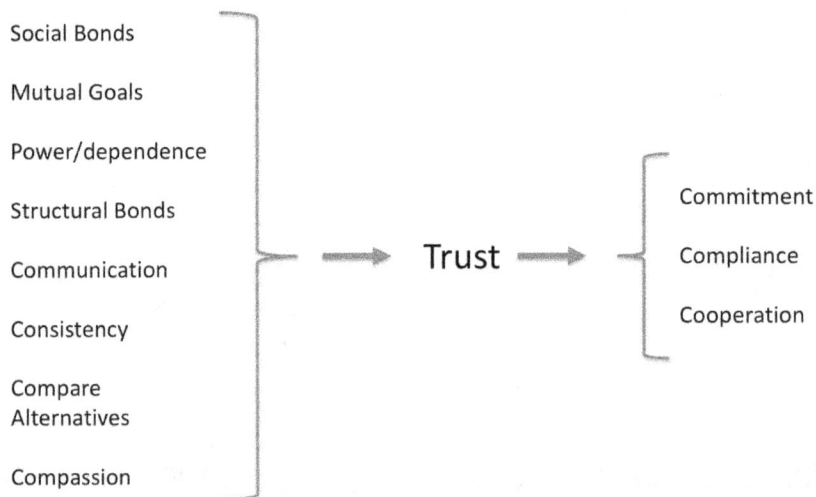

TABLE 4-1. Relationship Building Blocks

Essentially, a strong relationship is built on trust. If you can't trust someone, how can you have a long-term relationship? How you build that trust is key to achieving commitment, compliance, and cooperation. These three "C's" represent the desired outcome.

Let's start on the left side Table 4-1.

Social bonds. The ice breaker in building a relationship is getting to know each other socially. This involves asking questions about their family, interests, hobbies, etc. You may find out how many children they have, where they went to school, if they like sports, and so on. It is also necessary to notice unspoken characteristics, such as the type of clothing worn, and if their office has pictures and paraphernalia on the wall or desk. These factors can help lead to future conversations. This social bonding will help with the next encounter. Keep in mind that the provider can ask a lot of questions, but so can the front desk staff and triage team. Make sure to note these social items in the EMR to help everyone in the office get to know the patient better.

Mutual goals. When building a relationship with someone, you need to know what is important to them, what they expect from the relationship, and what makes up their own personal goals. There is a purpose in all relationships based upon the expectation or goals that contribute to why the relationship exists in the first place. In a provider patient relationship, the mutual goal might be to get well or, at the very least, to have an improved quality of life. In a sales relationship (for example, when a patient needs surgery and there is a sell required), the mutual goal would be to reach agreement on the price, service, etc. of an item.

Power/dependence. Like it or not, there is not only a mutual aspect in any relationship, but also a power position. One of the individuals involved has control most of the time, but which individual this is may vary and change based upon circumstances. In the provider patient relationship, who has the power? Often it is the provider who is leading the Q & A portion of the visit and instructing the patient what needs to be done to achieve the mutual goal of getting well. However, the patient may be in the power position when it comes to talking about their needs initially, or in complying with the proposed care plan. This dynamic is in a constant state of flux with the advent of the internet, and the incredible amount of information that is now available to the patient. The patient may have their mind made up on the diagnosis and treatment plan prior to arrival, which begs questions who is in control, and how do you deal with it. The power position suggests that there is always one dependent on the other in a relationship. This also applies internally. A new employee is dependent upon their coach to learn, but later the coach is dependent upon the employee to perform their assigned duties. This is not a negative context, but a real role definition. If the power or dependence becomes too dominant, the context turns negative, and the relationship is destined for failure.

Structural bonds. Any organization has a structure, whether it is written as an organizational chart or not. This formal approach to a relationship is necessary to ensure that everyone knows where they fit, how the work with others, and to consistently fulfill the mission. There is also structure in the very nature of the provider patient relationship, with the provider as the assumed leader.

However, here is a good place to also point out that there are structured relationships that are informal. These will have the power/dependence aspect to them. Many times, these informal relationships are very beneficial, but they also can be a problem in the organization.

Communication. Enough said! Well, not really. None of the aspects of the relationship are possible without effective communication. There is a sender of the message, and a receiver - a talker, and a listener. Listening is an art that requires focus. Beyond the obvious verbal communication is the non-verbal, or body language, message. Asking questions of a patient, but looking at the computer screen, may send a message of dis-interest or not caring about what is being said. Crossing arms in a conversation may also be telling, implying you are closer off to the receiver. In the electronic world, capital letters are interpreted as screaming. It is difficult to really understand what someone is saying, or their intent, in an electronic communication. Many times, the non-verbal, facial expression, or the direct opportunity to ask for clarification is missing, which makes the communication process incomplete and ineffective.

Consistency. Without communication being consistent, there is no way to know what will happen next or what to expect. The key point here is that sending a message that is authentic, and doing it regularly, will help build the relationship with the other party.

Compare alternatives. There are over 7 billion people on earth, and therefore there are alternatives. In some case it is best to choose the alternative, and in other cases it is best to recognize that there are alternatives, but that what you have is the right one. This concept becomes very important to remember for the provider and the entire staff of the practice. The patient has a choice, and if the relationship is not built on all the points above, the alternative will be chosen. There is always another applicant for a position. The alternative concept should be in the forefront of your mind in developing a relationship, especially with those who you serve.

Compassion. Compassion is defined as sympathetic consciousness of others' distress together with the desire to alleviate it. The patient is looking for a compassionate aspect of the relationship. In most cases, the discussion about the patient's condition is one requiring an understanding, as well as offering support.

Trust. There are many other terms that could be used, but I believe these are the basic building blocks leading to a level of trust. Webster defines trust as "assured reliance on the character, ability, strength, or truth of someone or something."[3] The basis of any relationship, then, is built on the idea that we trust the other party. If you cannot trust someone, how can you have a positive relationship? You may not trust someone and still have a relationship, but it will not lead to any of the three "C's."

The right side of Table 4-1 suggests that the outcome of all the above is a commitment to the relationship. The business and the individual expect and desires the long-term commitment. After all, it is easier, and cheaper, to maintain a relationship than it is to build one. A committed relationship will also benefit as a compliant one. The provider will be able to offer a better relationship, and achieve mutual goals, if there is compliance with the agreed upon care plan. This means there is full cooperation on the part of everyone, including the patient's commitment that the prescription is refilled timely to ensure health is achieved. As we look at the future of healthcare, the patient compliance to the treatment plan is essential. It may not be a valid "C" in the perspective of most relationships, but still worthwhile thinking about.

This is obvious when you think about the partner relationship or the employer/employee relationship. It is obvious when you consider the provider referral and the vendor/customer relationship. But as time moves forward, the need to build better relationships with the payers, the hospital "C" suite, other providers who may be competitors, employers, government officials – regulators or elected, and others that you may have in your local community.

The main message is the goal of approaching relationships in a structured manner, keeping these key concepts in mind.

Let's take a page from industry and apply it to our healthcare world. The manufacturer of a widget requires materials from others to complete construction. There may be one, or many, suppliers that require coordination and negotiation of items such as delivery time, amount, and price, information, and communication. This is referred to as a supply chain, where suppliers provide and meet the needs of the customer. Who has the power in this relationship, who benefits, and how do they benefit? In successful supply chains, all parties benefit from the relationship; this mutual partnership is key to each one's success.

A supply chain in healthcare may be as simple as patient to provider, or payer to provider. But in most cases, there are multiple players involved in meeting the needs of the ultimate customer. These include payer, hospital, clinic, equipment supplier, drug supplier, and many more. It is in this context that the individual practice lives and, hopefully, survives.

To accomplish this effort, there are three major barriers that must be overcome.

First to explore is the individual focus, beyond just the physician's role. Second is the tone of the organization itself, and the support structure in place to allow time and compensation to encourage involvement in tasks that are necessary for the organization to succeed. And finally, there is a need to understand the nuances of the outside world. This includes everything from the motivation of the partner, to the role and influence of government laws and regulations.

In today's population health value-based payment world, creating and maintaining partnerships that have common purpose, willingness to share data, and recognition that each member of the supply chain will benefit by working together, will lead to mutual wins. This requires open communication, understanding each other's goal, objectives, and needs, and the ability to work within those parameters. The openness required may mean joint planning meetings.

One can look at the payers with their emphasis on medical home models for both primary and specialty providers. They have significant data on the practice that they should be willing to share. The practice needs that data, along with their own data, to ensure that it accepts a payment level and quality metric level that is attainable. The payer must recognize the upper level providers and acknowledge that they are better off with those entities in their networks. A win-win is possible by being open to each other.

A partnership model might look something like what is noted in Table 4-2[4]

There are driving factors, or reasons, to enter the partnership, including a supportive environment, and the activities and processes that will make the relationship work. An important question to ask is if you drive or if others drive, and this perspective makes a difference in how you perceive the key aspects of the model.

Drivers with payer partners will include reimbursement amounts, quality metrics, contract termination terms, pre-authorization waivers, timely filing requirements, and other items. Drivers with suppliers will include pricing, rebates, delivery times and amounts, variety of products available, and the ability to contact the right person. Drivers with hospitals will include access to services, privileges, reporting, hospitalists, ED support, quality metrics, and information exchange.

A key point in developing partnerships is your identification of who you will choose as your partner. This is not just an external based decision. Rather, it starts internally. Multiple physicians have multiple opinions of products, hospital systems, referral sources, drugs, and

```
┌──────────────┐      ╱◇╲           ┌──────────────┐
│   Drivers    │    Decision to     │ Facilitators │
│  Compelling  │ →  create or    ←  │  Supportive  │
│ reasons to   │    adjust          │ environmental│
│   partner    │    partnerships    │  factors     │
│              │                    │ that enhance │
│              │                    │ partnership  │
│              │                    │   growth     │
└──────────────┘                    └──────────────┘
       ↓                                    
┌──────────────┐  ┌──────────────┐  ┌──────────────┐
│ Drivers set  │  │  Components   │  │  Feedback to:│
│ expectations │  │Joint activities│ │  • Drivers   │
│ of outcomes  │  │and processes  │  │ • Facilitators│
│              │  │that build     │  │ • Components │
│              │  │and sustain the│  │              │
│              │  │ partnership   │  │              │
└──────────────┘  └──────────────┘  └──────────────┘
       ↓                 ↓                 ↑
          ┌──────────────┐
          │  Outcomes     │
          │The extent to  │
          │which          │
          │performance    │
          │meets          │
          │expectations   │
          └──────────────┘
```

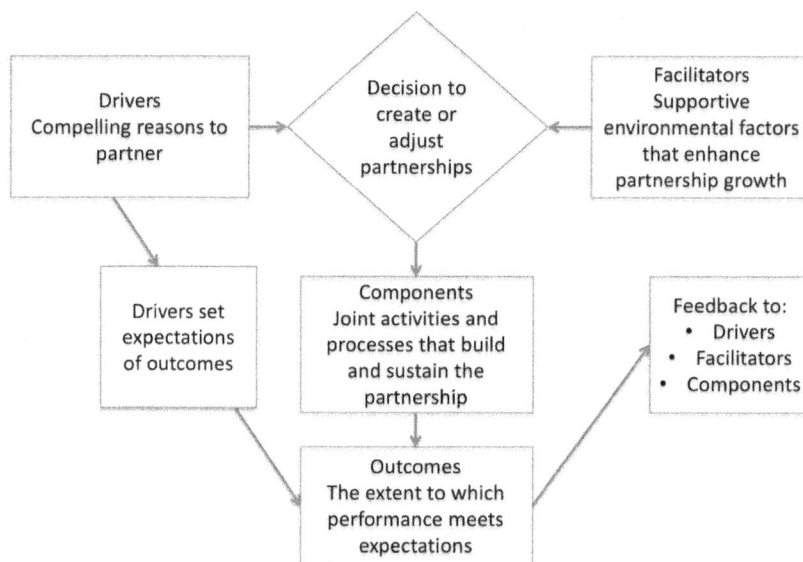

TABLE 4-2. Relationship Based Business Model

the like. Therefore, internal discussions will need to occur. Many hospitals face decisions on what knee joint replacement vendor should be used, as surgeons will have different opinions. This may not seem as big of a factor internal to the practice, but these discussions must occur. It is not advantageous to have two or three vendors for similar products. The practice is better off having the lengthy, difficult discussions internally before seeking a partner, rather than spending resources developing relationships only to have them fall apart due to lack of support internally.

Factors to consider reach beyond limiting vendors on supplies. One payer may consider a key procedure as experimental and have a long history of not supporting the innovative modeling that you do. Therefore, all other factors may be great, but a key procedure in your internal strategic plan may not be supported, or there are no plans for a payer to support that procedure.

A huge part of partnering is the relationship that is built on the key points highlighted in the Introduction. Obviously, you cannot have a successful partnership without a high level of trust with your partners. This is created with items like consistency, responsiveness, open communication, social norms, and much more.

How does your partner work? Digging deeper into who makes decisions, as well as when and how are they made, is a key to good working relationships. Neither partner has time to waste. If travel is an issue, can you communicate effectively via a digital model, or is face-to-face the best? Or better yet, what issues require face-to-face interaction? It is important that you are making appropriate plans for those communications to occur.

Supply and demand will play a big role. Does the payer offer a solid list of employers, or other patient sources? Who are the employers, and are you cut off from accessing them directly for wellness programs, etc.? Or is there a partnering way to achieve population health objectives?

Partners may best be chosen by recognition of, and/or elimination of the competition. The competitor may offer the same type and quality of service that you do but the employer base, geographic location, or other similar factors may make a relationship with a partner desirable.

The vendor must be able to provide products when needed, making it important to consider if they can be delivered the next day, or if delivery will always be delayed a few days. The demand for the supplies from the practice can be developed and managed on a "just in time" model. The "time" can be defined differently, such as next day or two days. Very few applications in the office would require same day. But delivery is critical, since it directly affects the amount of inventory the practice must have on hand, and reduces the funds tied up in inventory. Historical data, and the use of predictive analytical tools, will assist the vendor in their understanding of what is needed. This then reduces pressure on the vendor in managing their production and/or inventory needs.

Drug reps, and drug company, relationships are semi-restricted due to sunshine laws. However, the practice must question if their partner drug reps bring value in terms of clear understanding of the efficacy of the drug they are representing. Is a visit to the practice the only way that information can be obtained, or are there other options? Or, is this simply a way for the staff to get a free breakfast, or lunch? From a non-physician outlook, I can only assume that it still is critical to stay on top of the latest developments in drugs.

Does your practice have an established research program? There is a clear need to partner with drug companies and other sources of research projects. Auditors will visit the practice regularly, and it is important to be open with them, providing access to the documentation they require, in order to work toward a successful research program.

Medicare and payers have significant information on the practice. In fact, they may have more data and more of an understanding of the practice in terms of patient management than you do! HEDIS, payer Star programs, and core quality measure through separate programs and are excellent. HEDIS is designed to help payers and their programs, meeting five domains of care. They are not measuring what the payer does, but what the provider does for the payer patient population. The Star programs are for payers as well. The more physicians understand, and the more the payers and physicians work together, the stronger the network will be. Would the patient like to belong to a 3-star of 5-star network? The need to understand and work together with the payers is critical for the success of the practice. Think in terms of federal government programs, from PQRS to MACRA measure processes. Hopefully soon this data will become available and used for outcomes. The key here is the need to partner with Medicare and payers. They are part of the supply chain.

In many cases, the relationship with payers is antagonistic, rather than attempting to establish mutual goals and benefits. A revisit of this focus is in order. It is not necessarily with all payers, but certainly with the key payers in your practice.

Diving deeper, we identify another real benefit of partnering is the evolution and application of new ideas. We can learn a lot more from other industries. Keep an open mind, join the Chamber of Commerce, or other organizations that will expose you to the ideas of others. If a partner brings an idea to the practice, it is critical to be open to reviewing it. The idea may not work, but discouraging partners from developing new ideas, or not listening when one is presented, will have a negative impact on the relationship.

COMMUNICATION

What's missing in this chapter is an exploration of how effectively all parties communicate. Communication is key, and multi-faceted aspect of the supply chain. There is the sender, the message, and the receiver. How the message is sent, whether via email, in person, written, or other, is up to the sender. The method is critical to the success of the effort.

The internet is full of comments regarding communication, with the most interesting one citing a three-part breakdown. This breakdown is as follows:[5]

- 55% of the communication is body language
- 38% of the communication is tone of voice
- 7% of the communication is the words that are used

It should not be assumed that this only applies only to face-to-face efforts. Consider the receptionist who is having a bad day and answers the phone with a gruff voice and an attitude. An unwelcome message comes across loud and clear, even when it is delivered over the phone. Or the email that comes in all CAPS! If we are to effectively communicate, awareness of these three aspects is critical in all forms of communication.

So, how do we make communication work? Follow these steps:

- Identify your partners, specifically those who are in the supply chain.
  - Remember that there may be a direct line, e.g., payer and practice. But there also may be others in the chain such as the hospital, the vendor, the patient, other providers who will assist in the care delivery
- Arrange a meeting, or meetings, to work to reach agreement on expectations.
  - This does not necessarily need to be with all, but start with the most immediate contact and work from there
  - Establish mutual goals
- Develop an action plan for each party, and for the joint effort.
  - Identify action items
  - Establish priorities and milestones

– Agree on timelines
– Assign and accept responsibility
- Develop agreement to formalize all efforts.
  – Rules of the process
  – Formalize action plans
- Regularly review progress.
  – Regular time frame to meet
  – Be open and honest about the benefits or issues
- Revise process and agreement as necessary.
  – If agreed to continue, revisions may be necessary
  – Implement changes
  – Revise agreement
  – Agree on next review period

This framework applies to any and all efforts related to the supply chain partnership.

REFERENCES

1. Evariant. What is Physician Engagement? http://www.evariant.com/faq/what-is-physician-engagement. Accessed December 1, 2018

2. Wilson, DT. An Integrated Model of Buyer-Seller Relationships, *Journal of Academy of Marketing Science*, 1995; 23(4):335-345.

3. http://www.merriam-webster.com/dictionary/trust. Accessed December 1, 2018

4. Supply Chain Digital 4 Keys to Successful Supply Chain Implementation June 2, 2015; https://scm-institute.org/relationship-based-business-model/partnerships-in-the-supply-chain/. Accessed December 1, 2018.

5. Thompson J. Is Nonverbal Communication a Numbers Game? www.psychologytoday.com/us/blog/beyond-words/201109/is-nonverbal-communication-numbers-game. Accessed December 1, 2018

SUPPLY CHAIN PARTNER CHECKLIST

Understanding of the business environment	• Identifying the market characteristics of each product/service with the following:
	  – Customer needs
	  – Pressures from suppliers
	  – The level of competitor activity
	• Undertaking SWOT analysis to better understand the business environment and your current position on the market

Making analysis of the business	• Analyze and summarize the existing competence of the business • Define which operations are the core to the business and which ones can be outsourced • Gather the essential information on customer needs • Set strategic priorities to determine key areas of the business where supply chain management succeeds • Analyze the current situation with the supply chain to identify suppliers, customers and relationships with them

Examining the existing supplier base	• Compose a list of the suppliers for each product/service
	• Assess each of the suppliers against the performance criteria as follows:
	  – Price
	  – Reliability and responsiveness
	  – Delivery
	  – Quality level
	  – Product specification
	• Sift out suppliers with the poorest performance
	• Try to have as less as possible supplier base. The reasons are :
	  – Lower administrative costs
	  – More time to manage each supplier
	  – Better cooperation between the company and the supplier

Dividing suppliers into several categories	Divide supplier by groups such as "Under performing", "Preferred" and "Strategic"
	
	Work at each of the groups to reach cost reductions in the supply chain:
	  • "Under performing". These suppliers bring few improvement ideas to the supply chain
	  • "Preferred" . Negotiate with these suppliers to discover the potential to reduce handling, distribution and warehousing costs
	  • "Strategic". These suppliers are committed to found a long-term partnership

Establishing the supply chain partnership	• Build partnership considering the following conditions:
	  – Shared risk and mutual trust
	  – Mutual strategic interests and synergy
	  – Sharing privileged or confidential information
	  – Suppliers are involved in the designing of a new product
	• Start with a supplier the company already has good relationships with
	• When negotiating with a supplier, consider the following actions:
	  – Find mutual cost benefits (win/win scenario)
	  – Encourage ideas of benefit to both parties
	  – Base relationships on mutual trust
	  – Ensure the partner in long-term cooperation

Establishing the supply chain network with a process map	• Widen the established partnership to involve new customers and suppliers • Design a process map for the entire supply chain • Identify total costs and movements with this map • Use the process map to reveal areas of potential wastage
Monitor the supply chain	• Ensure that supply chain operates as planned and provides the benefits to all involved parties • Ensure that indicators and measures are monitored on a regular basis • React immediately to any shortcomings or delays through the indicators

Source: http://paksupplychain.blogspot.com/2011/05/checklist-managing-supply-chain.html

Chapter 5

Yes, Your Healthcare Practice is a Business

Whether or not recognized by physicians, the medical practice is a business. The quicker this is understood, the quicker your practice will begin to operate as a business. There are several key principles that define a business. A business must have a plan, a purpose, management, employees, a sound financial model, and customers. We'll talk about these in the sections that follow.

How healthy is your business? This is not intended to be a play on words, but instead, intended to help you focus on how well you and your business are doing. Is your business in good health, or would you classify it as sick? Using this physician mind set, consider the SOAP model of looking at the health of your organization. McKinsey and Company define organizational health as "the organization's ability to align around a common vision, execute against the vision effectively, and renew itself through innovation and creative thinking."[1] You should keep this definition in mind as we work through exploring the health of your business.

A PLAN

When coming up with a plan, you need to strategically ask questions like: who you will serve, what will you do, and how will you do it. This sounds simple, but it requires all owners of the business to be on the same page. It's not as simple as we will practice general surgery. It requires hospital or ambulatory care centers, scope of services –location of office, hours office will be open for patient visits, EHR, seeing Medicare patients, how many surgeons, are physician extenders needed, what skill level of employee in the office, and so much more. You get the idea.

To start, consider a strategic plan that realistically looks at the long-term perspective for your practice. Typically, this is developed at a planning retreat with the physicians, and lay leaders. It can be facilitated by an experienced consultant or lead by internal staff - whichever works best for you. These are best done when the participants are free from interruptions. These retreats can run for a half day, or up to two days, depending upon where, when, and the extent of the agenda.

The agenda should review items like the practice's strengths, weaknesses, opportunities and threats, and a thorough SWOT analysis. Openness in the discussion, leading questions, and a desire to create a unified look at the future is essential.

SCENARIO PLANNING

We have found, given today's uncertain environment, that the use of scenario planning is beneficial. A scenario plan considers alternatives for the future, and does not, necessarily, lay out one option. The fact that there are many external pressures identified in your SWOT (uncertainties at the federal, state, and local level) makes having different options key. This concept suggests that you consider four, or more, different scenarios that may occur over the next few years. Many think that a plan should have only one outcome, which can force a rebellion against the idea. But realistically, you can look at scenario planning as a way of better preparing for the future by considering multiple outcomes.

Scenario planning involves consideration for different approaches to the future. With the evolution of the Triple Aim, population health, value-based payments, integration of behavior health, and more, it may be impossible to choose one best scenario for your future.

Ask all participants to approach the process with an open mind. Brainstorming on ideas will lead to more creative insights and bring in more knowledge from each participant's perspective on the environment – both internal and external. By brainstorming, there will be more possible scenarios considered. This eliminates group think, where one, or a small group of individuals, create or control the plan and future. Doing so will be beneficial to the final strategic plan.

In setting the tone for this process you will want to:
- Identify events that are certain to occur
- Identify uncertainties, as well
- Be open to a broad range of possible outcomes for the future
- Encourage creativity, which will include some extreme ideas (which in a period of time may not be extreme!)
- To encourage openness, don't discourage, or reject, an idea immediately - keep all items open for discussion and thought
- There is no such thing as a stupid question or idea
- Be aware that there may not be enough data to substantiate a scenario
- Assume that today's best plan may not work tomorrow

In scenario planning, you create a matrix with four quadrants, with the X axis as growth, and the Y axis as stability. The lower left is the most conservative scenario, with the upper right being the ideal. The lower left may suggest that staying the same is a viable scenario.

The upper right may suggest taking leadership in expanding, or creating, a new organization, e.g., a physician controlled ACO. Use catchy names to identify each to help with future communications. The scenario considered most likely then forms the base of operations. The beauty of using scenarios is that, as things change, you will begin to see which scenario is most likely to occur. An important step to include in the process is to do some detail thinking and planning related to each quadrant. This is not a waste of time. Rather, it creates an awareness of what is necessary to achieve that scenario. Your annual plan, then, will consider what things can be done without favoring one over the other. Your annual plan will not negatively impact any one of the scenarios. You will not waste resources in your daily operations. You will have thought through each one, leaving you better prepared to act, when the time is right.

The next step is to create a business plan for the year, which seeks to implement key aspects of the strategic plan, while adapting a budget. It is not required that this occur at the strategic planning retreat, but must be part of the annual schedule of events. This not only includes the development and approval, but also acceptance and monitoring for the entire 12 month applicable period.[2]

One comment worth emphasizing here is the concept of "short-term-ism." The stock market is built on monthly, or quarterly, data and dividend distribution to the stock holders. The focus is immediate, or very short term. Many medical practices suffer from this same perspective. An example of this is feeling the need to distribute all funds at year end to avoid taxes. This can cause a narrow focus on what is best for the future. It also emphasizes activities at year end, which generate revenues. These activities may, or may not, be in the best interest of the patient or the community. The patient may desire a procedure since they have met their annual deductible, and do not want their care to pass on to the next year's deductible. This is not to imply bad or unnecessary care, but instead, to point out that any plan must have a focus greater than three, or 12 months.

A PURPOSE

This may sound redundant to the idea of the plan, but it is not. There are different motivations to run a business. Sometimes, the owners are not on the same page, with one wanting to make a significant income, while another puts the customer (patient) first, and is not as concerned about funding. This is why the purpose is identified as a key principle. The purpose should be stated in the mission statement.

A mission statement describes an intersection of what the environment is for your practice, and what your practice does to meet the needs of the customer, employees, and owners. This statement needs to be short, concise, and carry a true description to each of the stakeholders identified.

The mission statement answers four key questions. This should be simple, but requires all to participate, agree, and believe in the words used.

1. What do you do? Beyond simply providing quality medical care, be specific.
2. How do you do it? Your infrastructure, tools; principles applied to the processes.
3. To whom do you do it for? Identify the voice of the customer – what do they want, expect, and need?
4. What value to you bring to those served, your community, and yourself? Value and quality are interchangeable, how do you measure?

Consider some of these examples of mission statements:

From the Mayo Clinic web site, their mission statement:

"To inspire hope, and contribute to health and well-being by providing the best care to every patient through integrated clinical practice, education and research."

American Express mission states "We work hard every day to make American Express the world's most respected service brand." They follow with values. Your practice should consider similar statements to be included with each mission. Note the key words more than the expression.

Customer commitment – we develop relationships that make a positive difference in our customer's lives.

Quality – we provide outstanding products and unsurpassed service that, together, deliver premium value to our customers.

Integrity – we uphold the highest standards of integrity in all our actions.

Teamwork – we work together, across boundaries, to meet the needs of our customers and to help the company win.

Respect for people – we value our people, encourage their development and reward their performance.

Good citizenship – we are good citizens in the communities in which we live and work.

A will to win – we exhibit a strong will to win in the marketplace and in every aspect of our business.

Personal accountability – we are personally accountable for delivering on out commitments.[3]

To the scientific mind of the typical physician, words included in a mission statement, and in value statements, may seem like a waste of time. In management circles, these mean a lot. They send a message to the staff of what is important and what is expected. The bottom line, though, is once the words are in place, they must be upheld. Is there unity among all physicians, owners, and employees, to consistently live by what is openly expressed?

ORGANIZATIONAL STRUCTURE

Today's complex world will require an organizational structure that is agile, and yet can hold staff accountable for achievement of the goals set forth in the strategic plan. This is difficult, at best, when the culture of the organization is such that decisions are slow to be made, planning does not occur, and there is little - if any - effort to hold management accountable for outcomes (other than what the financial picture is at year-end).

What is your organization structure? There are many types, but here we will focus on three.

1. The traditional hierarchy with several levels of management include starting with the "C" suite of chief executives, directors, managers, supervisors, and lead workers, or some variance of the same. The areas of responsibility can be divided by division, e.g., ancillary service or geography. The other common option is to divide responsibility by function, such as front desk at several offices or nursing at several offices.

The traditional hierarchy has served its purpose, and works well in many situations. A word of caution, however, is found in one example where a healthcare system recently added several physician groups to the existing hospital. The hierarchy-based organization structure was revised, with a VP for physician practices who would report to the system President and CEO. Although seemingly positive, the VP was not allowed routine access to the CEO and was not comfortable bringing issues, big or small, for in-person discussion. This struggle, although possibly personality driven, could have resulted from the structure itself.

A change announced in late 2017 by Intermountain Health from geography or divisional reporting to one related to functional is interesting. The change is to create functional activity around primary care and secondary care roles regardless of locations. The feeling is this will reduce competition and better meet the needs of the patient. By no means is this a recommendation rather this is intended to suggest that any size organization can change to meet its perceived best approach to providing care to its patient population.

2. The second type is flat, or flatter, which reduces the number of titles in the hierarchy, and spreads the responsibility over more positions.

Both these types must consider the span of control How many managers should report to one director? Historically, it is thought that 7 or 8 is the maximum, as seen more often in the traditional hierarchy approach. The flatter organization will typically have more, in some instances up to 20. However, the number isn't as important as the director's attention and influence. The purpose of the reporting relationship isn't to focus on control, but instead the process or outcome. Some directors are not capable of a large span of control, or the work encourages a broad scope. The director will establish their team based upon their approach to management. Is control or development/ coaching important to the organization? Two-way communication will go a long way, and openness from all parties, will dictate the scope of reporting. Finally, the level of trust that is established between the director and managers is essential. With today's electronic communication and data gathering, as well as the level of complexity, the scope requires serious consideration into the extent of delegation of authority and responsibility.

3. The third type is a listed matrix, which is typically used for project management. The individuals identified are selected to assist with a project and will report to more than one person. This can create issues, like deciding who will do the evaluation, priority of work time and who controls the work schedule of the employee. The advantage is that the organization utilizes talent in many different ways to seek continuous improvement. The concept of utilizing project management is more common today. Being flexible, understanding the difficulties of management and reporting relationships, is essential. Project management training, for all levels of management, is beneficial to any healthcare organization.

As a follow up with the flatter organization structure and project management, leadership can choose to divide the direct reports into strategic and operational teams. This could look like one team focusing on long term thoughts and implications, while another could focus on operational issues. This encourages all to get involved and reduces the stress on the top manager to identify, and solve, all organizational issues.

As we look at today's environment with social media, and the opportunities that exist for stating opinions, influencing others, and crowd sourcing, a word of caution is in order. In an organization leadership, it is essential to ensure that the purpose, and the value achievement goal, is in place. If the team can run on its own, the result may not be in line with the practice's purpose. Matrix and flatter organization structures are positive, but they must be established and maintained within the confines of the organization itself.

One point of struggles for physicians in their organization is the role of board member vs. provider (employee). Decisions made, and actions taken, at the board level do impact what happens when in clinic. It is important to wear the right hat in the right environment. When fitting into the structure, remember the responsibility as a board member, and the impact of actions taken that must be followed the next day, or week, when in the clinic.

Is your practice one that focuses on the key objectives of innovation, customer first, followed by performance, and employee engagement? Considering this is essential, but you must explore whether your organization can respond to ever changing competition, value focus, and regulations through its organizational structure.

DECISION MAKING

Efficiency through an effective organizational structure will lead to a more effective model for decision making. In many physician practices, the decision-making process is encumbered by schedules. Because the medical world is ever changing, the need for efficient decision making is critical.

Decisions may be very routine, or highly complex. This suggests that decisions can, and should be made, at different levels of the organization. Figure 5-1 helps outline parameters within which decisions may be made.[4]

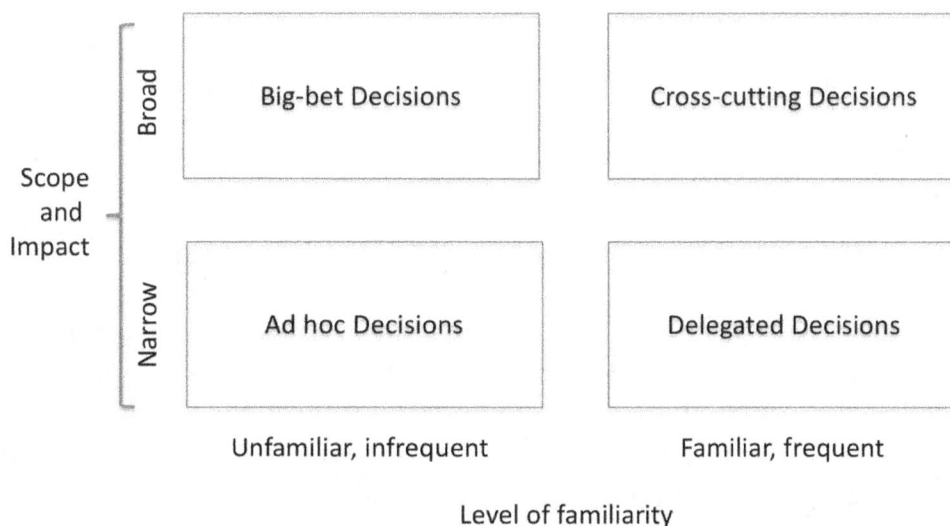

FIGURE 5-1. Decision Categories

Per figure –
- Big-bet decisions are infrequent and high risk, such as adding a new provider, opening a new office, or even closing an existing office. These are typically done by a select few with final decision at the board level.
- Cross-cutting decisions are frequent and high risk, such as adding a new ancillary service, negotiating a contract, or changing the fee schedule. These involve several different departments and staff members.
- Delegated decisions are frequent and low risk, and done within a department, within a budget, or within reasonable guidelines established. They do not need to be done at the board, or CEO, level.
- Ad hoc decisions are infrequent and low risk, such as changing vacation schedules within the department between providers.

These types of guidelines, when well thought out at the board level, will save time and reduce waste. Time is saved by knowing the details of the decision, and who will be involved in the decision. Waste is reduced in this aspect as well. Too often we find that decisions, big or ad hoc, are a major source of waste with no one knowing who should do what, when.

Another set of guidelines may be built on the amount of dollars involved.

Management can decide what amount of expenditures could be delegated to various levels of the organization. Even in flatter organizations, it may make sense to delegate. For example, the practice manager may be able to spend up to $1,000 without approval from the physician president or the board. Those who report to the manager may have up to $25 without approval of the manager. Even the receptionist could be delegated an approval of $40 for co-pay amounts, given parameters depending on the patient's individual case. Parameters of yes or no as a guideline can eliminate disruption from the work flow by giving the receptionist authority to make a decision on how to handle each patient, on any particular day.

MANAGEMENT AND LEADERSHIP

In all businesses there is a need for management and leadership. These are not the same. Many times, one physician has a clear vision coupled with a charismatic approach, getting others to follow. But the details required to make it work are not in their wheelhouse. This requires someone to who will manage the business. A leader sees that the right things are done to meet the purpose, and plan.

Alternatively, a manager will work with, and through, the human resources necessary to accomplish the desired purpose. This means effective utilization of all resources from staffing, to supplies, and inventory management. Financial knowledge is critical, but also is the ability to work with others.

The Picker Institute working with The Commonwealth Fund in a 2007 paper identified seven key factors related to achieving the goal of patient-centered (focused) care:[5]
- Leadership – commitment and engagement
- Strategic vision – clearly communicated
- Involvement of family and friends – care and involvement in the organizational structure and delivery
- Support for care givers – engage employees in design and delivery of care systems
- Measurement and feedback – continuous monitoring
- Quality environment – physical space and support
- Supportive technology – engage all directly in the care process

Each of the above points speak to where the current healthcare delivery system is headed, with a lot of work still to be done. It is important to review each of these key factors considering your current organization. Do you have these in mind as you approach your daily delivery of patient care? Is care in your organization focused to the benefit of the patient?

MOTIVATION

Why do you get up and go to work? What is it that gets you going, as you prepare for your day? Explore this one step further as a manager or leader of your organization. How would each employee in your organization answer those questions? What do you do, or what have you done, and what can you do move forward to motivate each employee in achieving your organization's vision?

Motivation as a management principle is traced back to Fredrick Winslow Taylor in the late 19th and early 20th century. He identified that workers could be better managed if four principles were followed:[6]

1. Replace basic work with methods based upon scientific study of what was required to do the work.
2. Scientifically identify, train and develop each worker rather than passively allow them to train themselves.
3. Cooperate with each worker to ensure that scientific methods are being followed.
4. Divide work equally (as possible) so each manager and worker had the same level of activity, allowing the application of scientific principles.

He suggested that time studies, incentive payments, and with equal application of work, there would be less fear on the part of the workers for losing their jobs if they became too efficient. These principles were key up until the early 1930's, however many of the key points still remain today about time studies, incentive plans, standardization, and elimination of waste.

An interesting study occurred in 1929 at Hawthorne Works, in Chicago. Elton Mayo set up two groups of employees. One was the control group, the other was given special treatment, such as better lighting, air circulation, etc. The goal was to see if these items improved productivity among the workers of that group. The findings revealed that both groups improved production. The outcome was that, not only did improved working conditions have a positive impact, but simply paying attention to others improved productivity.[7]

The Hawthorne studies and other efforts lead to new theories with the next major approach one of human relations management. Leading theorist here were Abraham Maslow (Figure 5-2)[8], Douglas McGregor (Figure 5-3)[9], and Frederick Herzberg (Table 5-1)[10].

As you consider Hawthorne and others, keep in mind two major factors: extrinsic and intrinsic approaches to motivation. Extrinsic are external to the employee, such as money, gift cards, increases to 401K, and the like. Intrinsic are internal, such as the employee contributing to the mission/purpose in some meaningful, satisfying way. Both are critical, but are not universal, for each employee and specific circumstances.

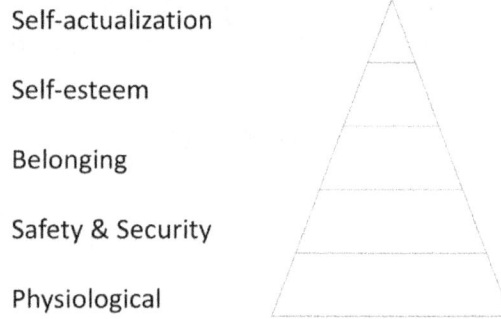

FIGURE 5-2. Maslow Human Relations Approach

Maslow's theory suggests that man has basic needs (such as food), safety needs (such as a place to live), belonging needs (being part of a team or group), esteem needs (others recognizing you), and finally, actualization needs, where you have achieved a high level of competence. You may switch between the need levels, but as lower needs are met, you continue to rise to the top level. Managers should be aware of all levels of needs, and work with employees to meet their individual needs.

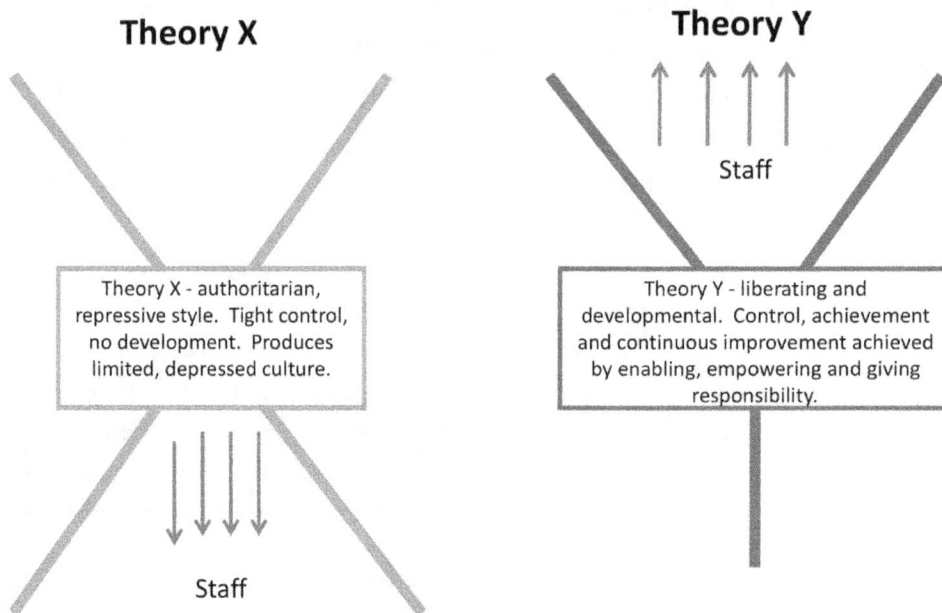

FIGURE 5-3. McGregor's Theory of Management

McGregor suggests that there are two types of workers. The first worker, Theory X, could always be classified as lazy and require direction, with tight controls on all work. Theory Y suggests that workers are self-motivated, willing to assume responsibility, and go the extra mile. The manager assumes one theory, and acts in that style regularly. An occasional need for the other style may surface, but typically workers fall into one category or the other.

TABLE 5-1. Herzberg Motivators

Hygiene Factors	Motivators
Company Policy	Achievement
Supervision	Recognition
Relationship with Boss	Work Itself
Work Conditions	Responsibility
Relationships with Peers	Growth

Herzberg suggests that hygiene factors are general areas, and that these alone will not motivate the individual to perform well. Instead, motivators are keys that will lead to improved production. Table 5-1.

Recently, Daniel Pink in his book, *Drive*, identified three levels of motivation.[11] His results are based upon a review of the history, as well as recent efforts to understand the world we live in.

- Motivation 1.0 – refers to Taylor's scientific management and Maslow's basic needs. Managers working in this area would approach employees related to structured processes, and that if basic needs are met they would perform well.
- Motivation 2.0 – refers to Taylor but emphasizes the need to recognize employee performance with incentives, and that if they are treated as humans, they will perform well.
- Motivation 3.0 – suggests that today's manager must go beyond incentives and rewards recognizing job performance. He expands the ideas of humanistic and suggests that involvement in tasks (training and education, coaching, and other ways to develop the individual) will lead to improved performance.

This is interesting as we remember that by 2020 approximately 50% of the work force will be Millennials. We discussed the generational and cultural aspects of people in the Chapter 3. Please review again, but put the tables in the context of employees, and how management should relate to each employee. Any motivational effort must be considered within the generational, and cultural perspective, of each employee. However, the context is just a guideline. Not everyone is the same, and there will be surprises. I recently had a discussion with a married couple who were both born in 1980. They considered themselves "tweeners" not really part of either the X or Y generation.

Given the shift in work force in terms of age, here are some helpful hints in managing the two larger generational groups:[12]

- Boomers have a job; millennials are looking for a career.

    Boomers have been in the same job/company most if not all their career. Millennials job hope, therefore, less sharing by boomers and loyalty from millennials will be the norm. Communicate clearly about the business and the opportunities to work toward retention.

- Millennials desire feedback, constantly, while boomers typically don't need it.

    The traditional annual evaluation is not enough for millennials, it is necessary to keep in mind the need to provide feedback, both positive and negative. The goal is career growth, contribution to the business, and work life balance – reassurance through transparency and effective communication.

- The challenges ahead are viewed differently.

    Millennials have multiple sources of income! They are looking at other things, the business should create opportunities, freedom for thinking about the future and better ways of doing things, can lead to retention.

- Boomers are OK with working, millennials want a work and live globally.

    It is much easier to travel both nationally and internationally. Millennials will not hesitate to make a move globally if the opportunity arises.

- Boomers know the business; millennials know digital.

    Social media, while we have heard a lot about privacy issues and advertising outreach, millennials are involved with digital activities. This can be both positive and negative. Create opportunities and use their talents to ensure a successful digital footprint for your business.

- TW^{2}ADI doesn't work for millennials.

    Boomers accept status quo (may not like it) while millennials do not.

Extrinsic motivational approaches may work for some, regardless of generational position, e.g., those on the lower levels of Maslow's hierarchy. Another example is in certain circumstances, such as improving collections over a short run for the revenue cycle team. Metrics that can be identified and tracked can lead to rewards, such as a bonus, dinner out with the group, or gift cards. Extrinsic rewards can work well for an individual occurrence also. One example is if a practice leader sees an employee diffuse a difficult situation with a complaining patient. The leader could approach the employee with a $5.00 gift card on the spot in front of other employees. It is not the amount, but the recognition of a job well done. It is important to reward behavior that is desired.

Intrinsic motivational approaches is a separate, more complex factor. This requires a culture, chemistry, and individual recognition. Let's use the earlier example. The employee who diffused the complaining patient may not need the gift card. Instead, they may have personal satisfaction by receiving a smile, or thank you, from the patient. By understanding the practice mission, values, and culture, the employee knew that treating the patient with respect was accepted and encouraged. They identified the right thing to do based on the training offered through the learning organization model. They were professional in their approach, and knew that they could tackle the issue.

MARKETING

We have purposely left the topic of marketing off the original list. It should be realized that all actions taken, based upon the information in this book, relate to marketing.

Simply put, marketing is creating an awareness in the market about your practice, and services provided to the public served. Marketing typically looks at what product/service is offered, the price charged (valid for payer relationships and private pay patients), promotion of the services identified, and where the services are best offered to meet the needs of the public served.

In today's world, the use of internet and social media is key, especially to the younger generation. However, all generations and culture do understand the concept of quality service. Patients are looking for the quick fix of quality health care, but they are also looking at the experience that occurs. "Word of mouth" advertising, and the way they explain their experience, is still invaluable to the marketing of your practice.

As you think about marketing your healthcare practice, consider these points:
- Patient satisfaction and providing value to the consumer
- People providing service, engaging, recognizing the importance of providing service to the customer
- The business of medicine without a business-based approach will have no organization, no direction, and no outcome
- Partnering with others in the supply chain and community, working together to achieve a satisfied customer who receives value
- Being efficient and effective in meeting the needs, respecting the individual in the process
- Recognizing the need and appropriate utilization of technology to improve service to the consumer, to coordinate care provided, to educate and inform all about the benefits derived from seeing that practice or that physician
- The ability to transition to a new model

The one caveat is the need to recognize the competition, and what they are doing. There has been a significant rise in alternative delivery options for convenience for patients, such as retail clinics and urgent care centers which are competing with primary care providers. Specialists are competing with each other. Healthcare system mergers are creating competition. In the latter, we however may be seeing monopolies or oligopolies which limit competition. Internal to the practice services provided must be excellent, and an awareness of the competition will help sharpen the approach.

The above offers a road map, and hopefully many things to think about. But now, how do you look at the future within the parameters of the Triple Aim – access, quality, and cost? The first step takes us back to Chapter 1 and asks you to consider if you have a solid infrastructure. It is not uncommon that the failure of a practice to survive, or the motivating factor to sell to another group or to a health system, is the failure to effectively manage the practice.

Access is not tied just to location. It is tied to how efficient the scheduling system is, and how the daily flow of the office operates. If you gain one minute per visit, and see 20 plus patients a day, the 20 minute gain translates to one more patient seen. This is revenue generating, plus providing more opportunities to serve your customer.

The cost question is simple - understand your cost. It becomes complex because when government and payers talk about controlling cost, they refer to the practice top line, or revenue. We know the status of the revenue, but do you know how much it cost to see a patient, or offer a diagnostic test or treatment in your office? We will explore more on this in Chapter 8 on finances.

How do you balance the resources necessary to care for one patient, with you in the exam room, with the broader picture of caring for the population? How do you measure the cost associated with that decision with the goal of staying in business? And can this afford you the opportunity to continue to provide access at a reasonable cost?

The flow chart, Figure 5-4 helps lead through these questions to a decision. An organized, well thought out approach, will lead to the answers to the above questions.

Let's take a specific example that was mentioned related to the behavioral health needs of patients. The case was made that there is a need for improved behavioral health. How can your practice respond to that need?

First step is to consider your patient base. There are several patients that seem depressed. The community has issues with opioid use, increasing teen suicide, and the major employer has laid off several employees.

The community has a need that accompanies the individual need. As you develop the business case, the first set of questions is whether you have the needed resources, staff, and financial and physical resources (space, equipment, supplies). If you followed the recommendations in Chapter 1, you have reviewed and fixed your infrastructure. Now the goal is to determine if you have the specific resources to meet the needs identified.

Determine how you will go about meeting those needs. Consider looking at three alternatives. The first one is to *collaborate with* existing community resources. If you collaborate, you must exchange appropriate patient information and ensure the patient is getting care from a qualified behavioral health specialist.

The second alternative is to *co-locate*, since you have existing space that is not being used. There is still a need to exchange information, but this alternative gives you easier, and almost

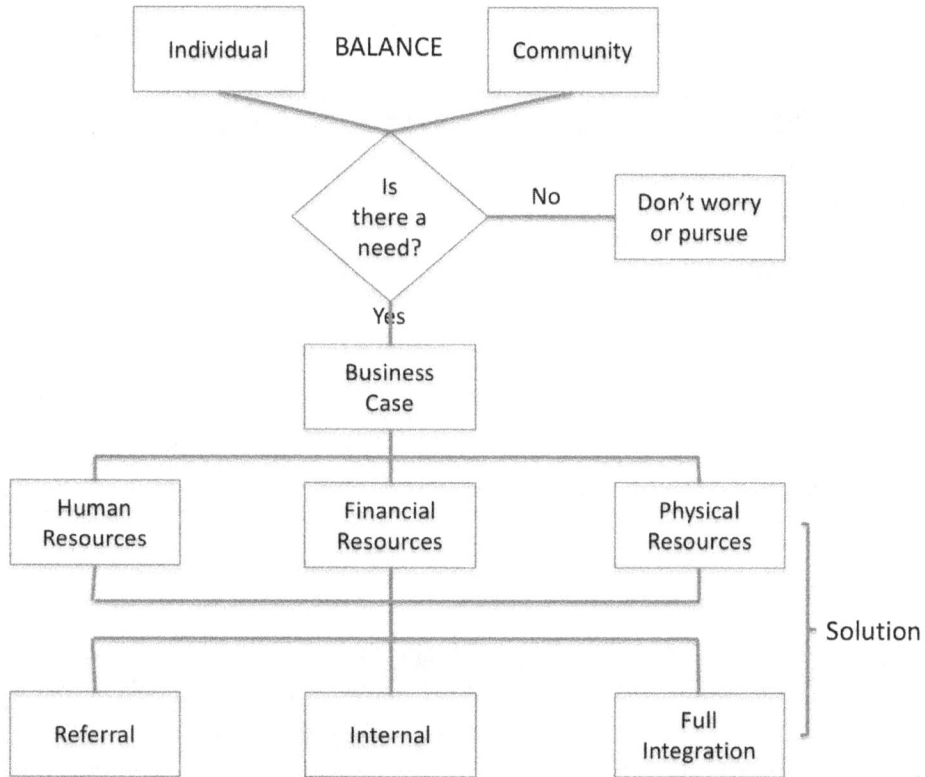

FIGURE 5-4. Managing Your Practice Within the Community

immediate, access to the specialist. This is comforting for the patient and helps finance your additional costs.

The final alternative is to *integrate* into your practice, meaning the specialist has ready access to all information, giving you immediate access to support for each patient. The exact level of support is optional, and open for review, as the plan develops as noted in Table 5-2.[13]

After reviewing the alternatives, you develop a strategy and business plan that starts with more formal collaboration, with the long-term goal of full integration. As you progress, you develop a secondary strategy which could involve reaching out to the school system, employers, city and county governments about how you can help. As they are open to the idea, you then develop an outreach program that includes education and counseling. This assures you meet the community need, but also expands your practice service lines.

Without a coordinated effort of all aspects discussed herein, there can be no business to provide service to the patient.

The practice leadership must accept that it is a business. Houston Methodist Healthcare System has a great saying, "The difference between practicing medicine and leading it."[14] Simply put, you are not only practicing medicine, you are the business of medicine.

TABLE 5-2. Integration into the Practice (Integrating Behavioral Health into the Medical Home: A Rapid Implementation Guide, 2016, Corso, et. al)

Job Title (Professional License)	Payment Level
Psychiatrist	100% of physician fee schedule
Clinical Psychologist	100% of physician fee schedule
Nurse Practitioner	85% of physician fee schedule
Physician Assistant	85% of physician fee schedule
Clinical Nurse Specialist	85% of physician fee schedule
Clinical Social Worker	75% of physician fee schedule
Licensed Professional Counselor	Not paid by insurance
Licensed Marriage and Family Therapist	Not paid by insurance

REFERENCES

1. Gagnon C, John E, Theunissen R. McKinsey Quarterly, Organizational Health: A Fast Track to Performance Improvement. September 2017, https://www.mckinsey.com/business-functions/organization/our-insights/organizational-health-a-fast-track-to-performance-improvement. Accessed December 1, 2018.

2. Roxburgh C. The Use and Abuse of Scenarios, November 2009. https://www.mckinsey.com/business-functions/strategy-and-corporate-finance/our-insights/the-use-and-abuse-of-scenarios. Accessed December 1, 2018.

3. Kolowich L. 17 Truly Inspiring Company Vision and Mission Statement Examples. https://blog.hubspot.com/marketing/inspiring-company-mission-statements. Accessed December 1, 2018.

4. DeSmet A, Lachey G, Weiss LM. Untangling Your Organization's Decision Making, June 2017, *McKinsey Quarterly*, http://www.mckinsey.com/business-functions/organization/our-insights/untangling-your-organizations-decision-making. Accessed December 1, 2018.

5. Shaller, D. Patient-Centered Care: What Does it Take? The Commonwealth Fund, October 1, 2007. https://www.commonwealthfund.org/publications/fund-reports/2007/oct/patient-centered-care-what-does-it-take. Accessed December 1, 2018.

6. Frederick Taylor and Scientific Management, NetMBA, http://www.netmba.com/mgmt/scientific/. Accessed December 1, 2018

7. Lumen Introduction to Business. Reading: The Hawthorne Studies. https://courses.lumenlearning.com/baycollege-introbusiness/chapter/video-hawthorne-studies-at-att/. Accessed December 1, 2018.

8. McLeod S. Maslow's Hierarchy of Needs. Simply Psychology; https://www.simplypsychology.org/maslow.html. Accessed December 1, 2018.

9. Dininni J. Management Theory of Douglas McGregor; February 22, 2017; https://www.business.com/articles/management-theory-of-douglas-mcgregor. Accessed December 1, 2018

10. Dininni J. Management Theory of Frederick Herzberg; February 22, 2017; https://www.business.com/articles/management-theory-of-frederick-herzberg/. Accessed December 1, 2018.

11. Pink D. *Drive*. New York, NY: Riverhead Book; 2009.

12. Boomer Millennial Harmony in 6 Steps. https://cdn2.hubspot.net/hubfs/2327869/PPL_WF/PPL_WF_HRCI_2018/HRCI%20-%20Boomer-Millennial%20Harmony%20in%206%20Steps.pdf?submissionGuid=c220e06b-b773-4f0c-9def-30791a60e766. Accessed September 1, 2018.

13. Corso K, Hunter C, Dahl O, Kallenberg G, Manson L. *Integrating Behavioral Health into the Medical Home: A Rapid Implementation Guide.* Phoenix, MD: Greenbranch Publishing; 2016.

14. https://www.houstonmethodist.org/. Accessed December 1, 2018.

STRATEGIC PLANNING RETREAT

Use the following questions to help you plan the retreat.

Purpose

1. What is the purpose of this retreat?
2. What criteria will you use to determine that the retreat was successful?

Participants

3. Who needs to attend the retreat?
4. Who supports the idea of holding a retreat?
5. Who is opposed to the idea?
6. Will all the key participants be able to attend?
7. How much time will they be willing to spend at the retreat?

Location

8. Where will the retreat be held?
9. Are the rules governing the use of the space acceptable?
10. Can the room be arranged as we want it?
11. Are the chairs comfortable?
12. Is there good control over lighting and HVAC?
13. Can we have food, snacks, and refreshments in the room?
14. Who will provide food, snacks, and refreshments?
15. Can we hang flip chart paper on the walls?
16. How will breaks and meals be handled?
17. Will overnight accommodations be needed?

Equipment

18. What equipment will be needed?
19. Who will provide it?
20. Who will operate it?

Facilitator

21. Do we need an outside facilitator?
22. Who will do it?
23. How much experience does the facilitator have with groups like ours?

Recording and Reporting

24. Do we want to record the meeting?
25. What kind of a retreat report we need?

http://www.ipspr.sc.edu/grs/A%20Guide%20to%20Planning%20and%20Conducting%20Successful%20Retreats.htm

MEETING MINUTES

For your regular monthly meetings, simplify you meeting minutes but ensure that all key actions are noted and followed up:

_____ (your practice name) _____Minutes

Topic	Discussion	Action to be/taken

ANNUAL BUSINESS PLAN AND BUDGET

Steps	Dates		Comments
	Start	End	
Review current performance against last year/current years targets			
Review SWOT			
Analyze successes and failures in this year			
Objectives for next year			
Identify resource changes necessary			
New budget for next year			
Accept plan and budget			
Develop review plan for next year			

COMPLIANCE OVERVIEW

Compliance plan:

- Written plan, reviewed annually and followed
- Compliance officer and committee, meet regularly
- Employee education
- Maintenance program for plan
- System to respond to inquiries and questions
- Audits of all systems
- Investigate, plan, correct, and re-evaluate

Major areas for review:

OSHA

- Exposure control plan
- Annual review and update
- Universal precautions
  - Biohazard warning labels
  - Hand wash facilities
  - Eye wash stations
  - Sharps disposal
  - Laundry
  - Trash containment and disposal
- Personal protective equipment
  - Gloves
  - Gowns
  - Makes
  - Eye shields
- Hepatitis B
- Post-exposure evaluation and follow up
- Labels and signage to communicate hazards
- Information and training for workers
- Employee health records
- OSHA 300 Log

HIPAA

- Business associate agreements
- Patient documentation
- Employee education

Fraud and Abuse
- Knowingly vs. mis-use
- False Claims Act
- Anti-kickback
- Physician self referral – Stark
- Criminal Health Care Fraud Statute

Clinical Laboratory Improvement Amendments
- Waived, PPM, APT
- Moderately complex
- Highly complex

Employment Laws
- Wage and Hour
- Age discrimination
- FMLA
- Sexual harassment
- COBRA

Chapter 6

Practice Efficiency, Lean Six Sigma, and Effectiveness

It goes without saying that any business can improve in its performance through meeting customer expectations. Simply look at your satisfaction survey results or talk to any patient who has been seen in your office, and they will tell you that things could improve. It is not something that will happen overnight. Rather, it is an attitude that starts with your acknowledgement of the need for improvement. Your new attitude is what jumpstarts improving your processes, and it leads to continuous process improvement, or CPI.

Much of what we will address is based on the principles in Lean and Six Sigma management approaches. These approaches originated from the manufacturing world. When discussing with physicians, there is a great deal of skepticism. Manufacturing uses assembly lines, and standardizes the pieces and parts used. Criticism has been that patients are all different, and thus the manufacturing process cannot be applied to the patient care process. This has been proven wrong.

Before we get into the more current thinking, let's reflect on one of the quality gurus who surfaced after World War II, W. Edwards Deming. An American, Deming helped Japan in its efforts to recover, and set into motion, many of the concepts found in the Toyota Production System - a key in the Lean movement.[1]

Deming identified 14 points that are included in the Deming Chain Reaction, depicted in Figure 6-1. Focusing on improving quality, flowing through the chain will lead to survival of your business.

His 14 points are all very valid, even today. Explore how each of these points is relevant to your practice today:

1. Create constancy of purpose for improvement of product and service –he follows Drucker's thinking that the mission is not intended to focus on money, but rather on the purpose to stay in business with innovation, research (on business models), and constant improvement. Serve the customer first.

2. Adopt the new philosophy – a religion where mistakes and negativism are unacceptable. No more waste (wait time), or medication errors, or unsafe environments.

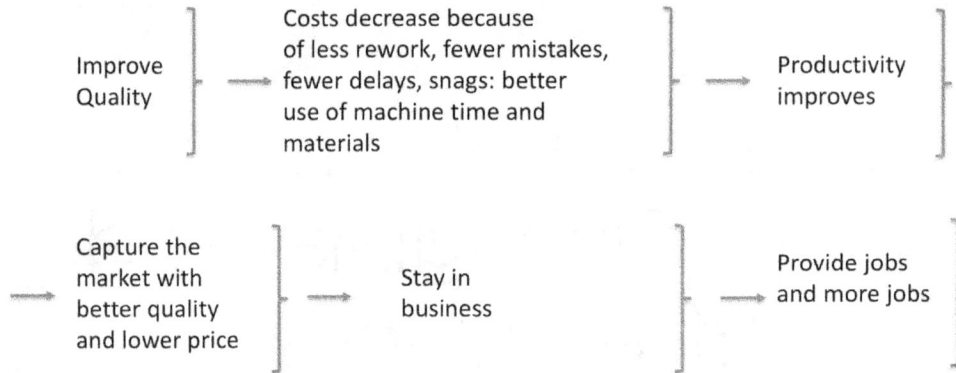

FIGURE 6-1. Deming Chain Reaction

3. Cease dependence on mass inspection – audits are great, but auditing everything, such as every charge entered into the practice management system, is a waste and unnecessary. Catching defects is costlier than not making them at all. Use audits as teachable moments.

4. End the practice of awarding business on price tag alone – a statement preceding value-based health care delivery.

5. Improve constantly. The system of production and service – continuous process improvement, is an improvement philosophy. It is not a onetime thing.

6. Institute training – create solid onboarding, along with individual and practice wide training programs.

7. Institute leadership – help staff do a better job through leadership and management improvement programs.

8. Drive out fear – employees are sometimes afraid to speak up for fear of losing their job.

9. Break down barriers between staff areas – those are the silos. Departments, other locations, even front desk and clinical areas often function on their own, rather than being part of the entire cycle of care.

10. Eliminate slogans, exhortations, and targets for the workforce – they simply don't motivate or help create an improved product, or service for the patient.

11. Eliminate numerical quotas – a quota is a number, not a method. Don't encourage staff to complete an arbitrary amount of work. Some are slower and struggle to do it, forgetting about quality over quantity, while others may be efficient and drag work out throughout the day or slack off once their quota has been met.

12. Remove barriers to pride of workmanship – faulty equipment, poor training, inadequate materials, and the like are barriers to success.

13. Institute a vigorous program of education and retraining – see chapter on the learning organization.

14. Act to accomplish the transformation – emphasis on the quality initiative, and that working together will lead to growth and success.

Deming also identified seven deadly sins:[2]

1. Lack of constancy of purpose, see number one above.
2. Emphasis on short-term profits – a narrow focus rather than a long-term perspective on where the practice is headed.
3. Evaluation of performance, merit rating, or annual review of performance. Yes, he categorizes this as a sin! The dreaded annual review that is not prepared well, and not received well, is a sin.
4. Mobility of management – this is particularly important with today's millennial work force. Develop management and recognize a job well done, continuously train and reward, retain key leaders.
5. Running a company on visible figures alone – make sure to look beyond the monthly financial statement. Big data gives much insight but be careful to make sure all data reviewed is meaningful and of value to the mission of the practice.
6. Excessive medical costs – this is from the perspective as an employer.
7. Excessive costs of warranty fueled by lawyers that work on contingency fees.

SIX SIGMA

The principle of Six Sigma is to eliminate defects from a system. The goal is simple: to achieve near perfection in doing any task. One example is medication errors; the frequency of prescription errors. Or, how many slips and falls have occurred due to errors, such as wet areas, rugs, or other things left on the floor? We will review tools that can help in the implementation of Six Sigma as part of our discussion below.

LEAN MANAGEMENT

Lean is an approach to management. It is built on many of the points made by Deming in his 14 points and seven deadly sins noted earlier.

- Lean is an approach built on solid, replicable metrics which form a base and reveal the results of your efforts.
- A Lean approach recognizes and seeks to eliminate waste.
- Lean respects the knowledge and input of people who do the work.
- Lean focuses on quality processes, and their safe application to your work environment.
- Lean is flow.
- Lean is a culture that seeks improvement in quality through a safe approach to the reduction of waste.

There are five principles of Lean:

1. Value – this is based on the concept that what you do, in your business, is to meet or exceed the expectations of your customers. Everything you do should add value to your customer. Your customer is willing to pay for value, but not for the waste associated with your service model.

2. Value stream – identification of the activities in your process that result in waste must be eliminated. How do you know what those wastes are? How you eliminate them is part of your analysis.

3. Flow – how smooth is your operation? How easy is if for your patient to move through your office with, no waste, in any step?

4. Pull – each step along the way of your process must tie together. When step one is complete, step two should be ready, and so on. If step two is not ready, then step one is may result in wait time and waste. The process should allow for a smooth flow, with each step ready when the previous step is complete.

5. Perfection – constantly strive for perfection by seeking continuous process improvement.

The main point is that value can be understood through the efforts noted in our discussion on patient satisfaction. However, it is important to realize that this point emphasizes customer. When reviewing process cycles for value, consider all who act as your customer. The patient is not your only customer. Any relationship that you have may be considered a customer relationship, even with payers. Also realize that fellow employees, referral sources, suppliers, hospitals and systems, and anyone in this context should be recognized as a customer.

Just as the patient is not the only customer, practice leadership is not the only one who can improve efficiency. This effort starts with you, but does not end, or rely, solely on you. It is essential to have a team to make it happen. Team members and roles include:

- Champion – this is typically a physician, or member of the "C" suite. While not directly involved with the project, this role signs off approval and offers support throughout the project life. Typically, this is a cheerleader role. Key here is the support of a physician, since physician-to-physician is the best way gain practice wide support and lead to the important culture change. This role acknowledges that there is a need, and a way, to improve.

- Leader – sometimes referred to as project manager, this role is the leader of the team. The work here is demanding yet rewarding. The business case, charter, team member selection, agenda, tool selection/implementation, and overall task master are key aspects of this role. The leader should have knowledge and experience in Lean Six Sigma principles, and keep the team focused on the scope of the project at hand.

- Process owners – these are the team members who do the work in the project being reviewed. Managing the front desk would include receptionists, not necessarily medical assistants (unless cross trained). These are the team members that know the extent of the work, how the work flows, and are very capable of coming up with new and better ways of doing things. Often in larger organizations, the director chooses the manager of the area to be on the team. This defeats the goal and role of process owner, so instead, reach to the ones that do the work to insure appropriate and implementable changes are identified.

- Subject matter experts, SME – these are folks that have knowledge which supports the goals of the project but aren't necessarily the process owners. These may include the information technology team, revenue cycle staff (if evaluating the front desk activity), and the like. They will participate with the team, but not necessarily attend all the meetings. They can contribute to the development of flow charts, cause and effect diagrams and the like.

- Facilitator – occasionally there is a need for outside assistance in guiding the team through the project. A social worker, trained in group dynamics, or a higher-level Black Belt, to guide the team leader may be a real benefit to the overall process.

- Recorder – it is essential to record all activities undertaken by the team. This memorializes the process, and tracks what worked and what didn't work. The documentation becomes critical in assisting the next project manager in managing their project. Eventually, the practice would gain a key guidebook of experiences, reducing waste and redundancy.

The Medical Group Management Association, MGMA, offers a series of training programs including White, Yellow, and Green belt for leaders and those interested in developing lean programs. A recent green belt participant had this to say about the points just made about team work:

> "I am truly amazed at how eager our staff is to participate in this process improvement project. We have physician buy-in, and inter-departmental collaboration the likes of which we have not seen before.... A long-time staff member who generally comes in, does the basics, and goes home has sprung to life! I asked for a Business Case in her words and was blown away by her response.... Not only are we effectively managing process change in a consistent manner within our practice, we are empowering staff at the same time. It is a beautiful thing to see!"[3]

The project life cycle noted in Figure 6-2 identifies the role and emphasis of the team members.[4]

The flow function could be reviewed with a key tool – a process map. The process map, or flow chart, creates a detailed breakdown of your cycle. Using pictures gives you a great look at how things work. These should be developed with a team of those who work in the process, the process owners. A simple way to create process maps is to use standard brown paper and affix to a wall. Ask your team members to identify on a sticky note what they

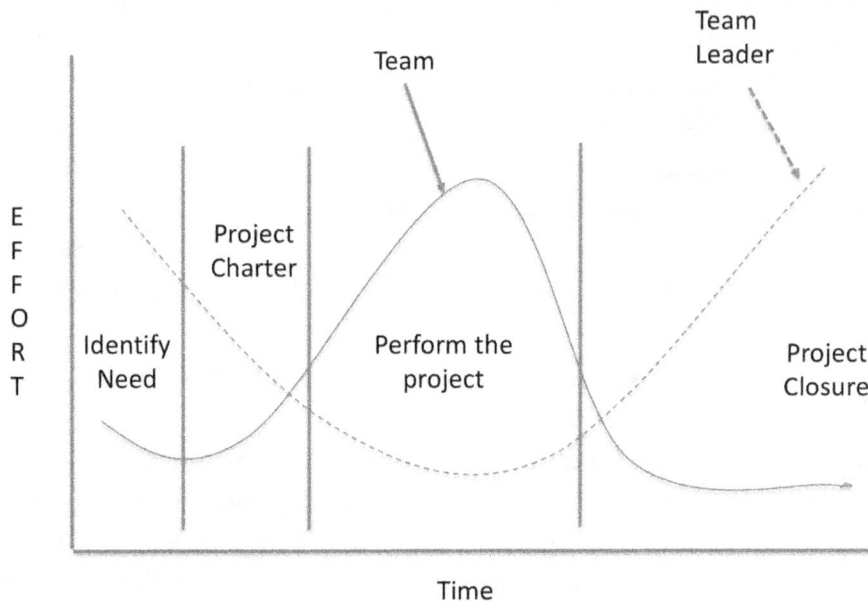

FIGURE 6-2. Project Life Cycle

do and ask that they be put on the brown paper in a sequence that follows their role in the cycle. If you have more than one process owner in the exercise, the task list and sequence will vary indicating some changes could be made to improve performance.

Process maps also use symbols, such as an oval for start, rectangle for process steps, and diamonds for decisions. In your brown paper exercise, use different color sticky notes for decision points in the cycle, and place them on a diamond angle, rather than as a rectangle. This creates a clear image of steps in the cycle. Again, it will reveal if there is a difference in what one process owner sees as a decision, and another does not. See Figure 6-3 for a quick look at a brown paper map.

This leads up to a key point related to the manufacturing process. A patient visit is a process which is continuous in its concept. It is repeated many times in a single clinic session. There is an amount of time that the patient spends in the process, referred to as cycle time. A legitimate question to ask each provider reading this is, "What is the average cycle time for your typical patient visit, a 99213 established patient?" If more than one provider is in the office, there will be a difference in that metric. This does not indicate that one is better than the other, yet simply points out that there will be a difference. This quick analysis of cycle time is what manufacturers do when looking at their assembly line. A patient visit is an assembly line. The goal of the manufacturer is to see where there are gaps and identify the barriers to the flow of the line. The analysis made by each provider is to identify similar gaps and barriers.

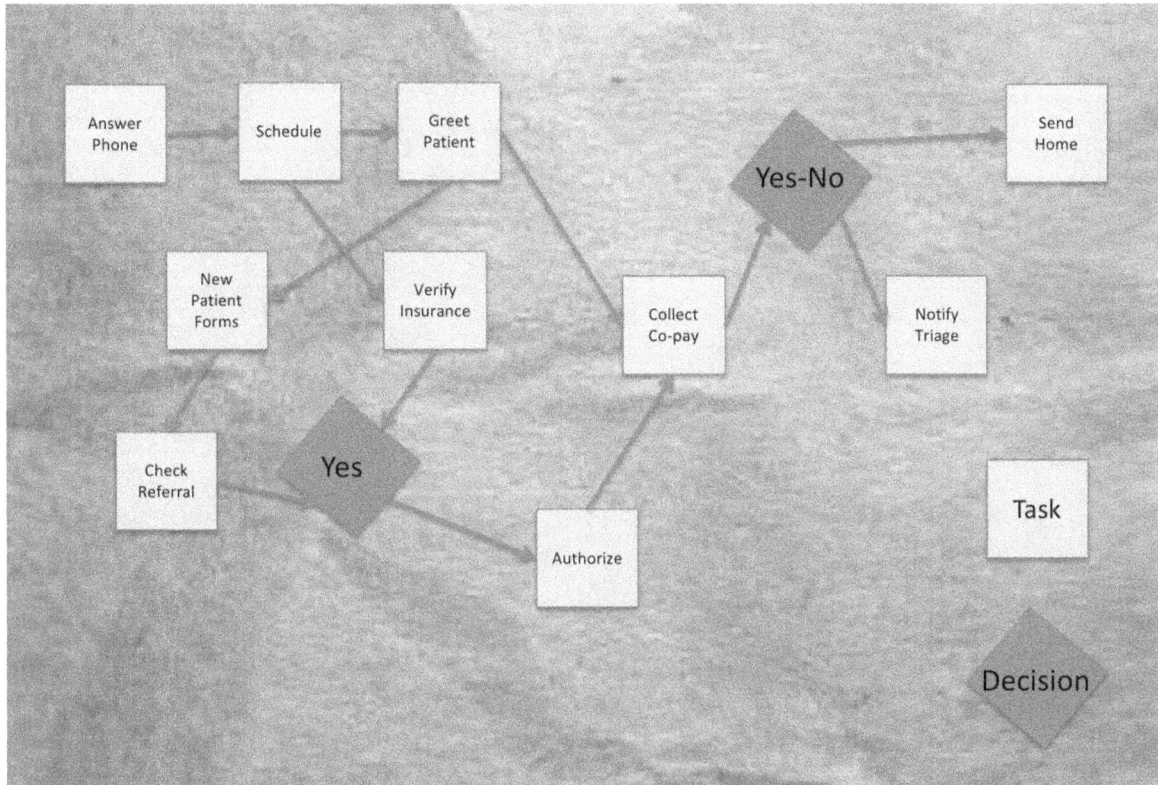

FIGURE 6-3. Brown Paper Process Map

The value stream, flow, and pull can now be looked at in some detail. Figure 6-4 offers a look at a patient cycle in two forms. The first, on the right, is a column chart noting the five key steps of any patient visit. There may be more for ancillary services but consider these five steps for the basic visit. The right-hand side is a process map with the symbols noted previously. They both illustrate a picture, but the column chart does is depicts a silo look, rather than a flow look. One of the keys in analyzing the patient cycle is to consider each step as related. The silo look implies that each piece is separate, and not necessarily related.

The value stream concept identifies what is of value to the patient, and what is "waste" in the cycle. Value in this case is defined as what the customer is willing to pay for, or what adds value. The customer is willing to pay for activities that relate directly to their care, but not the waste that is in the cycle. Non-value add is the time wasted waiting for interaction with the provider and team members. There is also business value add time, which is the time necessary for the business to function. The customer may not be willing to pay for this, but this time is necessary in the patient visit cycle.

In Figure 6-5, the total value add time is 25 minutes identified as triage, provider, and post activity. The non-value time is the time between value add and reception area is 26 minutes. The business value is 8 for a total of 59 minutes.

5 Steps in the Patient Cycle

Process Map

Silos

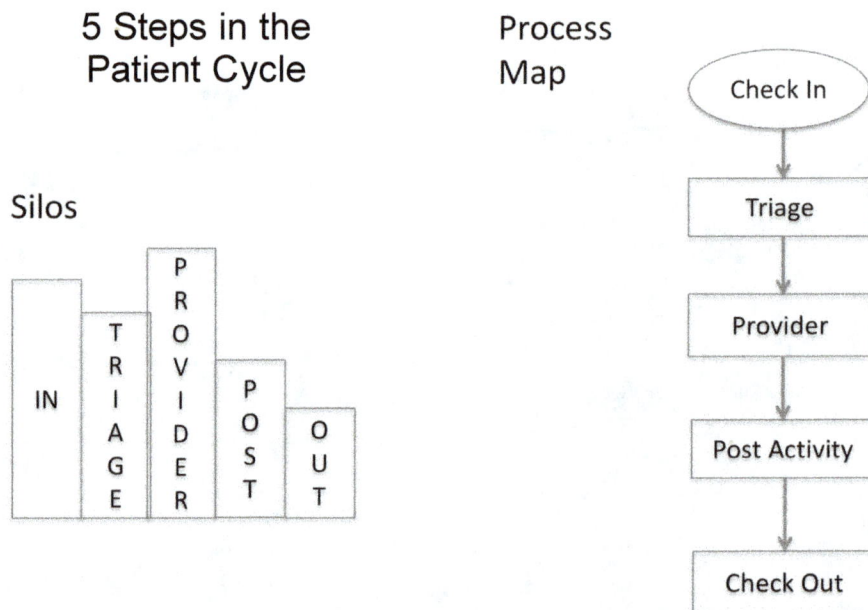

FIGURE 6-4. Two Looks at Patient Cycle

Another way to look at these numbers is to consider the efficiency of the cycle. In our example, the process cycle is inefficient since more than 50% of the total time the patient spends in the cycle is not bringing any value to them.

If we then look at the pull principle, we can see gaps between each value-added step. These gaps are not huge and may be necessary. It is important question this as it is unclear if all the non-value add time is necessary.

In reviewing the value stream cycle, we might look at value add first. If we can reduce time spent per patient for value-add components, we might be able to gain actual visit time, maybe even adding one more patient per day. The one more patient per day will result in increasing revenue, spreading fixed costs over more activity, and reducing the per visit cost.

So far, we have discussed efficiency. It is important to realize that this is not the only point to the patient cycle. There is also the need for effectiveness. There are exceptions for those patients that are not average, or typical. Effectiveness is important because there also needs to be adequate time to understand each patient need, and possibly the development of a more complex treatment plan.

One of the keys in analyzing the practice is to consider value, and non-value, of managing the cycle. A starting point in the analysis would be to look at activities around the provider contact. Are the tasks performed as business value add, or the supportive aspects of value add, done timely? Are they necessary, necessary at that time, or redundant to what the

Established Patient Visit

| Check In | → | Reception Area | → | Triage | → | Provider Time | → | Post Activity | → | Check Out |

| Demo Insurance Payment | | Vitals Reason RX check | Exam | Schedule Educate | Double check Schedule |

| 4 minutes | | 8 minutes | 12 minutes | 5 minutes | 4 minutes |

17 minutes   4 minutes   3 minutes   2 minutes

Process Cycle Efficiency:

25/59 = 42.4%

Total Time: 59
Value Add: 25
Business Value Add: 8
Non Value Add: 26

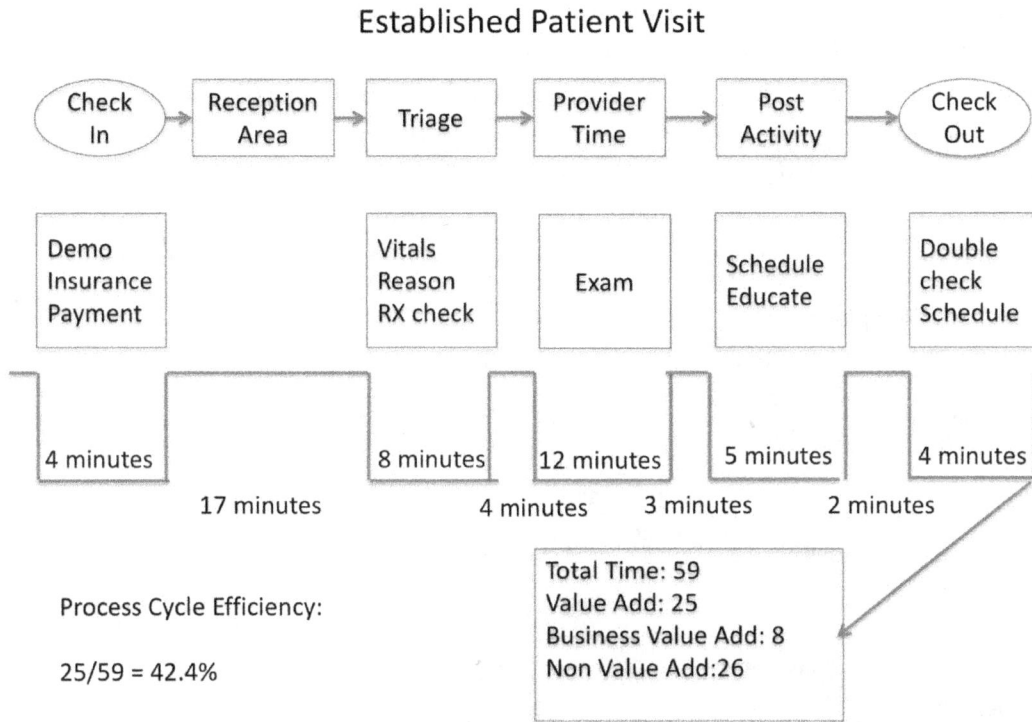

FIGURE 6-5. Value Stream Map

provider will do? The next step is to look at the non-value add time, or value add time that may be done more efficiently. This will then help create a more effective patient visit cycle, without first starting with the provider. The Lean principles can help the provider as well.

For example, another tool is 5S – where you always do everything to keep all things needed in their place. The 5S's are – sort, set in order, shine, standardize, and sustain. Apply these steps to each exam room, so the provider does not have to look around for anything. The provider will know it will always be in the same place, in each room. Each employee can use this for their own work area, for each supply closet, etc. This can save a few seconds, or few minutes, for the average patient visit, eliminating non-value add time and improving the effectiveness of the provider visit.

Let's also look at the role of triage. In the case management, value-based model, triage the patient's needs on the initial phone call can lead to the best option for delivery of care. This could be an immediate referral to an ED, a scheduled visit later that day to the office, or answering a routine question. Triage during the visit is also critical since this is where the necessary information is gathered for the provider. The provider can then focus on the real issues and will have a significant amount of information available to provide an efficient visit and adequate treatment plan, based on the best clinical guideline defined by the practice. Triage may be the most important role of any in the future.

A more detailed tool is the creation of a fishbone diagram, used to identify what causes lead to an outcome (Figure 6-6). This can also be referred to as a root cause analysis. As you analyze your cycles or defects found in the practice, this helps you identify what factors act as the root of the cause. Once recognized, a plan to repair or remove the cause can be created, resulting in a more effective outcome.

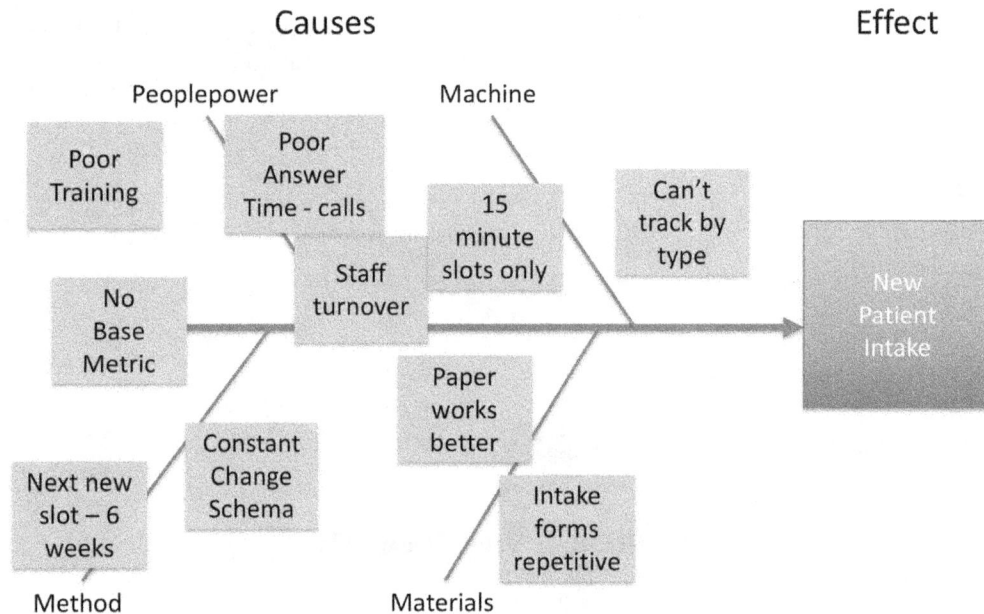

Causes   Effect

Peoplepower   Machine

Poor Training

Poor Answer Time - calls

15 minute slots only

Can't track by type

Staff turnover

No Base Metric

New Patient Intake

Paper works better

Constant Change Schema

Next new slot – 6 weeks

Intake forms repetitive

Method   Materials

FIGURE 6-6. Cause and Effect (Fishbone) Diagram

A very simple tool is to ask a staff member why they are doing an activity, or why they are doing it the way they choose. Typically, you may need to ask up to five times to get to the true answer. By the time you get through this exercise, you will find the cause. This is very simple, but effective, and can be done as soon as you see the next staff member doing something.

One of the keys to remember, as well, is that any improvement program starts at a recognition of the need to improve. But this does not always come from the top. Recognizing the skills of employees, and that they have incredible insights on how to make things better, is vital to jumpstarting change. The Japanese term Gemba means go to where the work is performed. Get out of your office and see what is happening. Experience the work environment and be open to what is happening.

When you consider a lean program, there must be buy in and acceptance from the top. This role is recognized as another type of team member - the Champion. A champion may be a physician or high-level executive. The champion may not be involved in each meeting but must be kept informed. The champion will help sell the idea and the solution to others. The champion is a key spokesperson, especially at the beginning.

At Toyota, they have an interesting approach to monitoring the assembly line. They have Andon cords throughout the plant. An Andon cord can be pulled by any employee. When pulled, it triggers alerts to supervisors that something is wrong. If the Andon cord is pulled hard, it stops the assembly line. Any assembly line employee in the billion-dollar business can halt production when they see something wrong. Would you be willing to stop your clinic session to review something that an employee senses are wrong (not life threatening)? Instead, encourage staff to be aware of issues, and give them sticky notes. Have an Andon board installed in the training area or break room? Sticky notes are placed there and are reviewed at the next daily huddle.

All these tools work by themselves. However, they are most effective when put in the context of a structured approach to improving the operation of the practice. This starts with the recognition, as noted above, that there is a need to improve the processes in the office. Leadership must buy into this and support the efforts, or the success rate will be marginal.

A more structured and managed approach, rather than one that is hit or miss, will bring the results desired. There are two optional deployment platforms that need to be considered. The first is DMAIC – define, measure, analyze, improve and control. The second is PDSA – plan, do, study, and act. The most common one used in Lean management is PDSA.

DMAIC suggests that step one is to define the issue at hand. This can be done after the use of one of the tools mentioned above or can be the starting point based on patient satisfaction survey results and any other source of problem identification. The measure phase is identifying a base line, and then further gathering data which offers additional data to enhance the review. The analyze phase reviews the data, identifies the root cause, brainstorms, and creates some ideas leading to a fix for the problem. Improve is implementation of the proposed solution. Finally, the control phase implements the solution and monitors it to ensure that it meets the expectations initially set out.

PDSA combines the first three parts of the DMAIC in the P phase. It moves to the do phase usually by doing a pilot study of the initial solution. The results of the pilot are studied and revised, as necessary. The act phase then is fully implemented and monitored.

Several key points to remember here:

- Defining the problem is difficult and requires time and soul searching. Too often, we all feel we know the problem and defining it is simple. Instead, it is possible that over time, the problem begins to creep (it grows as it is investigated and becomes big, yet nothing happens), or the scope broadens, and other problems are included. All this dilutes the real problem that needs to be addressed.

- When measuring or digging into the problem "project creep" can occur which means the scope of the problem grows and often gets to the point where is it so large that nothing gets done. Instead of project creep, keep your defined problem in focus and work on that. Pick the largest area where efforts to improve will have the biggest initial impact. Then in the last phase, review the project again and work on the next biggest area to fix. This is continuous process improvement!

- The need for a "champion" is essential. This role is typically one of the physicians who supports the need for improvement, is kept informed regularly of the efforts, and becomes a spokesperson for the solution, while promoting the idea that the practice needs to continually improve.

- The last stage, either control or act, is not the end of the project. Instead setting a time frame for review of the solution, looking at the next biggest area of impact, etc. is key. Just because the effort is complete does not mean that there is no longer need for further action. Accountability for the effort, for the staff implementation, and further measures will insure that the Lean program has been successful.

A key to any Lean or Six Sigma effort is to recognize that there will be failures along the way. It is possible to set a goal, identify a hypothesis at the beginning phase of the process, only to have the outcome not achieve anything, or even fail completely. Failure is a possible outcome for any venture However, the key from the perspective of these efforts is to try, learn from the attempt, and improve the next time.

The US Army has an excellent process, the Army After Action Review, AAAR. After every action undertaken by the Army, the key players assemble and review what went right, and what went wrong. It proves to be a great learning moment. Perhaps this concept could be adopted in your practice as well.

We have seen over the years many successes, but also many failures in the attempt to improve quality through the adoption of lean principles. Some examples:

- Credential process is more automated
- Redundancy in who does what in the patient visit cycle is eliminated, e.g., medical assistant and provider asking the same questions
- Location of supplies and equipment is streamlined
- Telephone call routing is enhanced, reducing delays and eliminating patient frustration
- Referral control for emergency department visits, better monitoring and control
- More complete, better timing on employee evaluations increasing performance
- Reduction in employee turnover through mentoring and coaching
- Inventory control programs, reduced cost of supplies and eliminated out dated stock
- Reducing registration paperwork for new patients
- Improve automation for scheduling, verifications, and authorizations

Congratulations to all those who succeed. The biggest reason for failure can be simplified to not enough time allocated to work through a change. When deciding to fix something, pick out a small project that leads to a win and positive results. Once the recognition that improvement is needed and that the process worked, another small step can take place. Keep working through until the philosophy is part of the culture. Time spent is worthwhile. So, work the process steps into the regular work day, and the results will amaze you.

Thus far, we have addressed a concept referred to by the Japanese as Kaizen, or continuous process improvement. The idea is that incremental fixes will over time result in gradually, and then drastic, improvements in outcomes for your customer. These are measured by improved profitability, improved clinical outcomes, or improved patient satisfaction scores. This is a philosophy that requires significant acceptance of the need of a culture change.

It is possible, however, to accept an approach advocated in the early 1990's by Michael Hammer and James Champy coined reengineering. This is not a Lean or Six Sigma approach using Kaizen, but rather a radical approach to completely changing the organization. The formal definition is "the fundamental rethinking and radial redesign of business processes to achieve dramatic improvements in critical, contemporary measures of performance, such as cost, quality, service, and speed."[5]

They identify four key words: fundamental, or looking at what a company must do, and how it must do it; radical, or getting to the root of things, while throwing away the old; dramatic, or quantum leaps in improved performance; and, processes, or a collection of inputs and outputs to achieve a revised, desired outcome.

They do make some key points that are worthwhile as you consider either a continuous process improvement, or a more radical reengineering approach to improving your patient care delivery. Some examples are:

- Combine several jobs into one, rather than handing some things off to others. This eliminates errors (waste) and miscommunication. How about the receptionist serving as the medical assistant, as well?
- Workers make decisions, which cannot be emphasized enough. The ones who do the work are the ones best suited to identify the solutions, and just as importantly, to implement the solution.
- Processes have multiple versions. As was discussed earlier with clinical guidelines, there may be two or three best options to consider when determining the course of treatment for the patient. This may also be the same in the management role. There are always alternatives to every decision. Determining which is best is the tough part.
- Work is performed where it makes the most sense. Is it right that the medical assistant schedule a routine revisit, or is that best left to the checkout staff, or an online application?
- If the work is done correctly by the right staff at the right time, continuous review, or checking on this, is redundant and a waste of time. Random reviews may be necessary, but correct reporting can also help identify if there are any gaps in the process.

It is not our point to suggest reengineering is the best option. In fact, it came into favor, and went out quickly. The important point is that, in some cases, a complete redo is necessary.

We prefer to think the key is the process. Don't focus on one project, or only one thing to fix. Instead, keep it going through a continuous process improvement program.

REFERENCES

1. Walton, M. *Deming Management at Work*, New York, NY, Pedigree Books by Putnam Publishing Group; 1991.
2. Walton, M. *Deming Management at Work*, New York, NY, Pedigree Books by Putnam Publishing Group; 1991.
3. E-mail correspondence; Director of Revenue Cycle, Orthopedic Specialty Group, E-mail March 12, 2018.
4. Cohen F, Dahl O. *Lean Six Sigma for The Medical Practice: Improving Profitability by Improving Processes.* Phoenix, MD: Greenbranch Publishing; 2010.
5. Hammer M, Champy J. *Reengineering the Corporation, A Manifesto for Business Revolution*, New York, NY: HarperCollins; 1993.

JOB DESCRIPTIONS FOR LEAN SIX SIGMA TEAM MEMBERS

Stakeholder:
- Sponsor who is actively involved in the project or whose interests may be positively or negatively affected by the project.
- Exert influence on the project.

Team champions:
- Upper level managers who control and allocate resources
- Have some training in process improvement techniques
- Lend support and encouragement from the practice upper level
- Involved in initial allocation of resources and support, involved in key milestone review points, and accept the project on behalf of the practice at its conclusion. (Final authority or recommend to final authority to accept project)

Team leader:
- Provide direction and identify assignments for tasks and time frames
- Act as liaison to upper level management
- Handle administrative duties, e.g., meeting site and times, task scheduling, milestone management, and the like
- Enforce meeting rules and regulations, manage team dynamics
- Work with and not over (or against) team members
- Encourager

Process owner:
- An expert regarding the process being reviewed or studied
- Knows the process inside and out
- Able to assist with process and value stream mapping – current and future state development
- Have an understanding of process improvement techniques
- Support team mission and goals
- The doer rather than the manager

Subject Matter Experts, SME:
- Offer expertise in a particular or technical area
- May be fellow employees or someone from outside the practice
- Good communicator, may be "geek" in nature but knowledge brought is key

Recorder:

- Records key activities – agenda, minutes, and updates throughout the project
- Follows guidelines per the project guidebook or practice model

Facilitator:

- Not really a team member!
- Outside team structure who brings skills at working with teams
- Understand group dynamics
- Understand the lean six sigma process to assist in keeping the momentum on track

For more details see: https://www.managementstudyguide.com/six-sigma-project-team-members.htm

PATIENT CYCLE TIME LOG

Monday   Doctor_____   Date _____

	DX (reason)	Check In	Check Out	Total Time
8:00				
9:00				
10:00				
11:00				
Noon				
1:00				
2:00				
3:00				
4:00				

Tuesday   Doctor_____   Date _____

	DX (reason)	Check In	Check Out	Total Time
8:00				
9:00				
10:00				
11:00				
Noon				
1:00				
2:00				
3:00				
4:00				

Wednesday   Doctor_____   Date _____

	DX (reason)	Check In	Check Out	Total Time
8:00				
9:00				
10:00				

11:00				
Noon				
1:00				
2:00				
3:00				
4:00				

Thursday   Doctor_____   Date _____

	DX (reason)	Check In	Check Out	Total Time
8:00				
9:00				
10:00				
11:00				
Noon				
1:00				
2:00				
3:00				
4:00				

Friday   Doctor_____   Date _____

	DX (reason)	Check In	Check Out	Total Time
8:00				
9:00				
10:00				
11:00				
Noon				
1:00				
2:00				
3:00				
4:00				

Instructions:
1. Identify first established patient visit per hour
2. Check in = is appointment time, not sign in or walk in
3. Check out = is when patient activity is complete for the visit
4. Record check in time in column
5. Record check out time in column
6. If no established patients seen in hour note None seen
7. Do not record new patients

MODEL FOR PDSA (PLAN, DO, STUDY, ACT) DEPLOYMENT PLATFORM

Use this as a model for the deployment platform, PDSA:

Telephone Management: Problem (opportunity):
1. Appointments
2. Prescription refills
3. Test results
4. Provider call back to patient/family

Plan:

- How would you define or identify your biggest problem (opportunity)
- What tools would you use
- How long would you measure, what amount of data would you want
- Can you measure, how would you – electronically, manually
- Who would be on the team
- What is you expectation, hypothesis

Do

- Implement test solution
- How long
- Where, who, how

Study

- How did you do, meet hypothesis
- What changes need to be made
- Next step, pilot again or role out

Act

- Implement full program
- Identify strategy for next phase or next project

Chapter 7

Instill the Culture of a Learning Organization

From the moment we were born, we began the lifelong process of learning. As a child, we learned by observing, listening, and experiencing. We were open to all things new. As we grow, our experiences begin to take form through what we learned, and what we did. The knowledge gained shapes us into who we are today. Consider how you learn, now that you are grown. Do you learn just for yourself, or for you chosen career path, or for growth in another area? This chapter explores what can be done to help you learn within your organization to help meet its vision, as well as to improve you as a person.

In 1990, Peter Senge wrote his bestselling book, *The Fifth Discipline*, which defined the concept of a learning organization.[1] His five disciplines offered a framework to create and operate in a learning environment. These disciplines are:

- **Shared vision** – the organization has a purpose and vision that it strives to achieve. This vision should be shared with all in the organization.

- **Mental models** – our experiences shape how we think, and what we do. How we react, and why we do things the way we do, are based on our mental models. The big issue in a learning organization is to understand everyone's mental model and how best to help those individuals learn. Employees are different based upon their age, their culture, the ethnicity, and so on. This is not a negative, but rather an important fact to keep in mind as leaders and managers consider their learning organization.

- **Team** – each learning organization has teams that need to work together to contribute to the vision of the organization. These are not silos; these are not departments with a purpose and function entirely on their own. Individual departments do exist, but there is a need for organizations to relate one team (department) to another. Individuals learn, but so do teams. How the organization addresses team learning is crucial to its success.

- **Personal mastery** – how can the organization help individuals achieve mastery within themselves? This speaks to personal growth in areas related to their teams and responsibilities, but also to their own improvement. A lifelong learning process will help all achieve a level of mastery in their chosen profession, or area of interest.

- **Systems thinking** – putting the previous four disciplines together in the system will achieve the vision. By putting this system together, one hopes to improve patient care for all served.

In today's complex medical world, the need to respond, to improve, to change, and to innovate is based on the need to learn. *Here we suggest that a learning program, rather than a training program, become a cornerstone for success in your organization.* In some ways, this may seem like a play on words, but the concept here is not to train, but to encourage learning for all members of the organization. Through learning, the organization will be better able to respond to the constantly changing world. This learning program may have several aspects, but two key ones should be operational and clinical. The outcomes should be improved patient care and a solid financial performance for the organization. Training helps identify the 'how,' 'what,' and 'when' that is necessary for growth. But learning offers the 'why' behind the training.

LEARNING ORGANIZATION MODEL

The learning organization model:

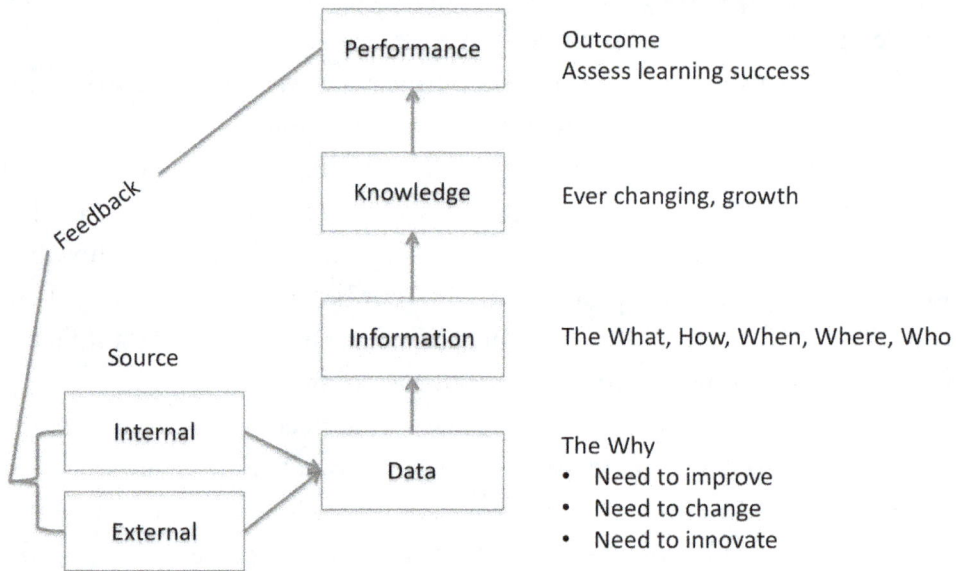

FIGURE 7-1.

Start at the bottom of Figure 7-1. What data do you have, what data is available, and what can you do with it? Data comes from external sources, such as what the competition is doing, what is happening in the local market, and what others are doing (benchmarking) to succeed. Internal sources come from your practice management system, EHR, and your financial management system.

This data will help compare your performance to your goals, and your key performance indicators. KPI relates to your outcomes. Once you identify the data that is relevant to your vision, you can then identify areas to improve or change. You also can be encouraged to innovate. After exploring the data, you may realize the way you've always done it no longer works to meet the goals of the organization.

This data gathering then helps focus on what information needs to be shared, or rather the 'what' piece of the equation. The 'how,' 'when,' 'where,' and 'who' will lead to the creation of the learning program.

The performance will then be measured against the goals and KPI established through the data review. This is then fed back to the base phase of the learning organization for a focus on continuous improvement and growth.

GOALS

Any program developed must have goals, or a purpose for its existence, and a way to measure its success. Each organization will need its own set of goals, here are a few:

- Change your culture to one that focuses on learning as an everyday, every activity component
- Improve performance
  - Employee development and retention
  - Enhance skills and capabilities
  - Achieve engagement of team members and patients
  - Meet KPI
- Achieve compliance
  - Regulatory requirements
  - Internal policy and procedures
  - Care/treatment plan
  - Ethical approach, no fraud, no abuse
- Develop and manage a succession plan
  - Identify key positions that require someone to take over
- Increase innovation
  - Do not accept the standard way as the mantra. Instead, challenge each member to find ways to improve what they are doing.

Here's a list of possible benefits from a learning organization:
- Superior performance and competitive advantage
- For customer relations

- To avoid decline
- To improve quality
- To understand risks and diversity more deeply
- For innovation
- For our personal and spiritual well being
- To increase our ability to manage change
- For understanding
- For an energized and committed work force
- To expand boundaries
- To engage in community
- For independence and liberty
- For awareness of the critical nature of interdependence
- Because the times demand it
- The main benefits are;
  - Maintaining levels of innovation and remaining competitive
  - Being better placed to respond to external pressures
  - Having the knowledge to better link resources to customer needs
  - Improving quality of outputs at all levels.
  - Improving corporate image by becoming more people oriented
  - Increasing the pace of change within the organization
- Even with, or without a learning organization, problems can stall the process of learning, or cause it.
- Because of these global trends, the value of human capital is even greater now than ever before
- Knowledge of key personnel within the organization can be made explicit, codified in manuals, and incorporated into new products and processes
- Leads to responsible decision making through knowledge. Allows for educated choices.[2]

What would you place as priorities on your list?

ADULT LEARNING

As adults, we are at a different stage in our learning process. We have gone through many stages, and methods, of learning.

Learning styles relate to using skills through vision, auditory, or kinesthetic. Consider if you were to ask a team member a question about their experience at a recent event. Make sure to listen closely to their response. If they use "I saw ..." or "the graphics...," they are more visual in their learning approach. If they use "I heard..." or "the music was great...," they are more auditory. Of if they respond with "I felt..." or "enjoyed the experience...," they are more kinesthetic. As you approach a team member, you should recognize their dominant learning approach in mentoring, coaching, or formal training.

One of the key points in the LO model is mental models. Malcom Knowles has identified key principles in adult learning that must be considered in the development of any learning program.[3]

1. **Self-Concept**

   As a person matures his/her self-concept moves from one of being a dependent personality toward one of being a self-directed human being.

2. **Adult Learner Experience**

   As a person matures, he/she accumulates a growing reservoir of experience that becomes an increasing resource for learning.

3. **Readiness to Learn**

   As a person matures his/her readiness to learn becomes oriented increasingly to the developmental tasks of his/her social roles.

4. **Orientation to Learning**

   As a person matures his/her time perspective changes from one of postponed application of knowledge to immediacy of application. As a result, his/her orientation toward learning shifts from one of subject- centeredness to one of problem centeredness.

5. **Motivation to Learn**

   As a person matures the motivation to learn is internal.

Given this list, consider the fact that each employee is different. There are different cultures that are not only formed from experience, but also relate to how and what is important to them.

GENERATIONS

We have covered generational differences, in general, in other sections of this book. If traditionalists and boomers are set in their ways, we will focus on the Gen X and Y generations in terms of developing approaches for them.

The Florida Institute of Technology has put together an excellent review of traits and strategies.[4]

Generation X Learner Traits

- Unlike the typically idealistic Baby Boomers, Generation X tends to be skeptical and cynical
- Independent and self-reliant
- Entrepreneurial thinkers
- Resourceful / problem solvers
- Defy authority
- Reject the "pay your dues" mentality

- Loyal to individuals, not organizations
- Reality driven: how will training help them in the real world?
- Have a distaste for "touchy feely" teaching methods
- Competent with technology
- Intolerant of bureaucracy
- Value freedom as the best reward
- Multi-taskers / balance work and life

Instructional Strategies for Generation X Learners
- Offer direct / immediate communication (Emails and phones)
- Get to the point and provide clear instructions
- Avoid micromanaging them
- Make assignments "real world"
- Provide opportunity for individual work
- Incorporate technology when possible
- Use games and case studies

Generation Y Learner Traits
- Tend to be optimists
- Expects immediate feedback
- Not accustomed to negative feedback
- Short attention span
- Wired 24/7
- More accepting of authority than Gen X
- Sheltered (by their helicopter parents)
- Team oriented
- Strong sense of entitlement
- Highly visual learners
- Expects accommodations
- As digital natives, they expect technology
- Often concerned with style over substance
- Opinionated

Instructional Strategies of Generation Y Learners
- Gen Y likes to communicate through texting and social media
- Provide clear objectives and standards
- Develop self-assessment items
- Provide opportunities for group work
- Incorporate technology
- Create a multimedia environment

- Offer chances to multi-task
- Give them group projects to complete
- Connect to learners through social media (Edmodo is great for educational purposes)

Once again, be cautious in the use of these points since they are general in nature, there may be "tweeners," and not everyone will fit into the category specifically. The strategies noted here are excellent when considering the development of a learning program for the younger team members.

EMOTIONAL INTELLIGENCE

Daniel Goleman published his book on emotional intelligence in 1995. His acronym is EQ. This concept suggests that the IQ, intelligence quotient, of an individual is only part of the person. He highlights five domains of EQ:[5]

1. Self-awareness - Knowing your emotions
2. Self-regulation - Managing your own emotions
3. Motivation - Motivating yourself
4. Empathy - Recognizing and understanding other people's emotions
5. Social skill - Managing relationships

There is a dark side to emotional intelligence, as well. When working with your team, be aware of the group think idea, or that one employee may be strong in their ability to sway others to their way of thinking. Extreme examples of strong emotional leaders include Adolf Hitler. Not to say that an employee would be at that level but have caution as you consider the emotional state. Develop your training programs with the idea that the emotions of the team member are critical to the successful relationship, and compassionate approach to caring for patients.

APPROACHES TO THE LEARNING PROGRAM

What do you need to do to develop and design a training program for your practice? Figure 7-2 offers a framework:[6]

This should apply whether you are training everyone in the practice, such as annual OSHA training, or just training a new employee. If we look at each box noted in the figure, consider the following:

1. Needs assessment – what do you need to train? How critical is the need?
   a. Organization wide program to meet strategic or regulatory requirements?
   b. Operational in nature with skills and tasks requirements considered.
   c. Individual needs from onboarding to targeted skills or tasks in their key work area.

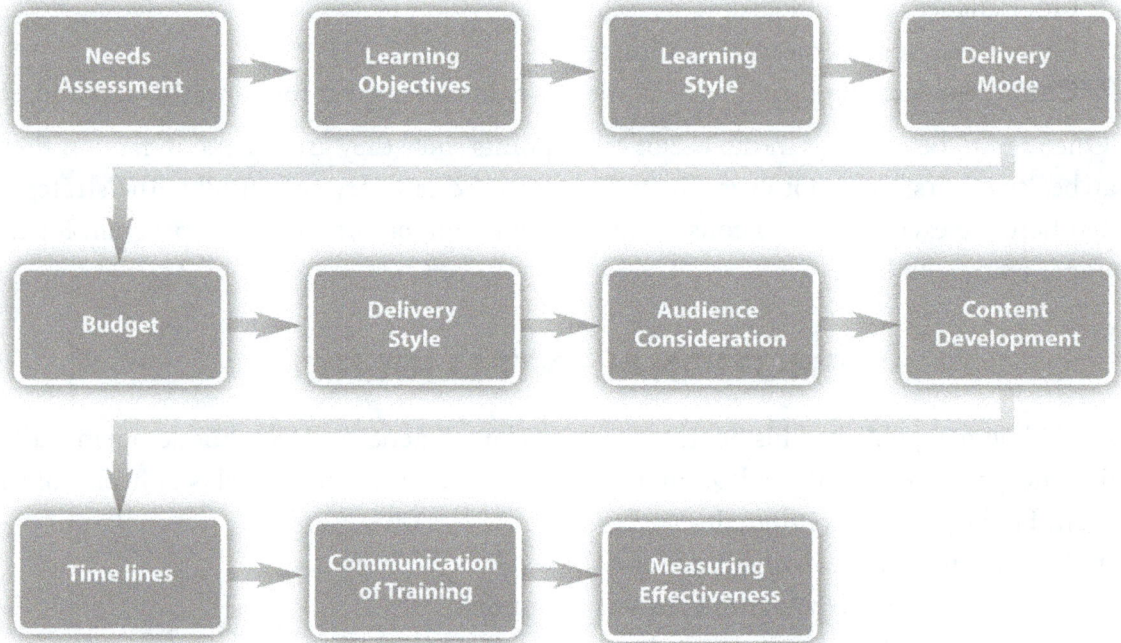

FIGURE 7-2. A Training Program

2. Objectives – what do you wish to accomplish with the training effort? What will the participant be able to do, explain, or demonstrate that they learned?

3. Learning style – each program or individual may require a specific training style or approach.

4. Delivery mode – classroom, eLearning, mentoring, or something different?

5. Budget - The cost benefit of any program effort must be considered.

6. Delivery style – formal, informal? Typically, the more interactive styles are better than a lecture format.

    a. Power point – but be cautious of 'death by power point,'

    b. Role play

    c. Case studies

7. Audience – to whom will the program be directed?

8. Content – based upon the needs assessment, what will be taught? Who will teach, and do we have resources in house, or do we look outside for help?

9. Timelines – when will the training occur, how long will it last, and how frequent will the program occur?

10. Communication – how will team members be made aware of the program?

11. Measure effectiveness – how will you know that it worked? What are the key metrics, or methods, to be used to ensure the program was successful?

Kirkpatrick offers a model for assessment[7]

a. Reaction – how did the participants react?

b. Learning – did the participant improve or change in their level of knowledge or skills?

c. Behavior – did the participants behavior improve or change in a positive direction?

d. Results – did the practice gain from the training effort?

Another key need that is often overlooked is the aspect of a succession plan. Very often the senior physician has been the practice leader (regardless of title) for many years, and the common perception is that they are invincible. Too often there is little done to develop a replacement, or a team of replacements. Beyond the lead physician, there are roles for other physicians, managers, skilled technologists, and mid-level providers. We can even look to the receptionist - do we have someone who can step in to do the tasks? What will it take to fill that unmet need, should it arise?

Additionally, don't forget the idea of cross training. This can result in cost saving, employee retention, and improved performance through the daily process. When more know, and understand, the requirements of related positions (e.g., front desk and billing office, front desk and scheduling), the more awareness of others' tasks and cross training will provide positive results.

When considering the objectives of any training program, the Bloom's taxonomy model works well. See the Figure 7-3.[8]

A formal classroom works well for certain types of messages, but this may be less likely to be successful today. Reaching many team members with required information is key. This may work well for regulatory learning. It is also important, though, to consider the approach used in the setting. Interactive learning options are better for adult learners. Instead of a power point lecture with the presenter off to the side, get interactive. Stand in front of, walk around, and reach out to the audience. Use role plays by getting members involved with specific identities to get the message across. Case studies given to small groups who attempt to solve the problem, and then present their findings to the entire audience, is a very viable option. The Socratic method of asking questions about the material, drilling down to get the entire message across, also works well.

E-learning options are a viable alternative. There are companies that have prepared programs that can be purchased for individual training. Topics include software, regulatory, and other technical programs.

One of the most effective approaches is to design and develop individualized programs through mentoring or coaching. Mentoring is when an individual (not the employee's direct report) is picked as a designated model for another employee. A key here is that the mentor does not provide all the answers, but rather works with the employee to help them find, or

Bloom's Taxonomy

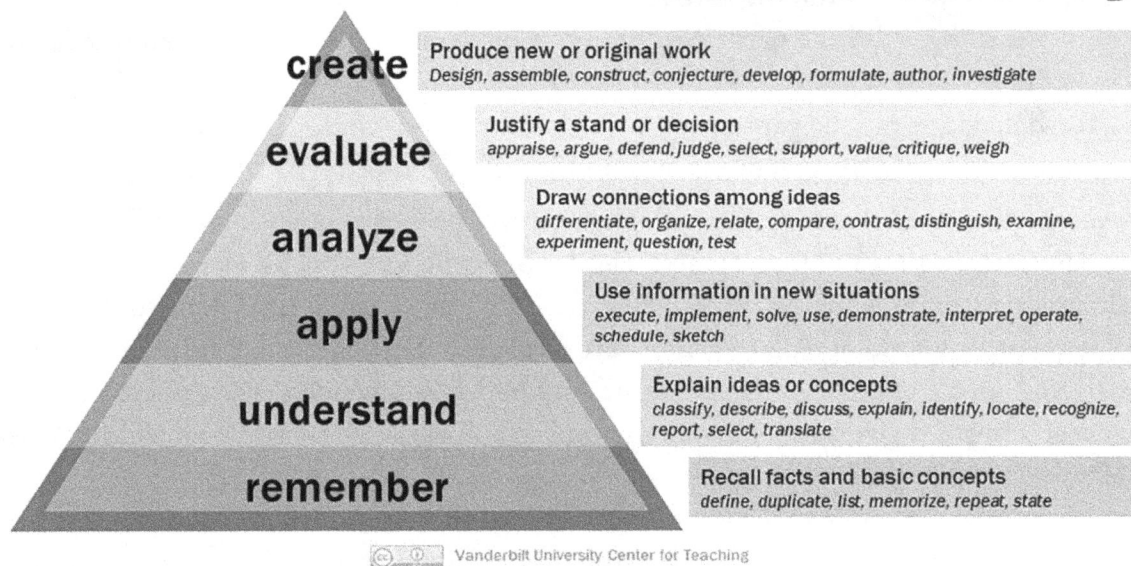

create — Produce new or original work
Design, assemble, construct, conjecture, develop, formulate, author, investigate

evaluate — Justify a stand or decision
appraise, argue, defend, judge, select, support, value, critique, weigh

analyze — Draw connections among ideas
differentiate, organize, relate, compare, contrast, distinguish, examine, experiment, question, test

apply — Use information in new situations
execute, implement, solve, use, demonstrate, interpret, operate, schedule, sketch

understand — Explain ideas or concepts
classify, describe, discuss, explain, identify, locate, recognize, report, select, translate

remember — Recall facts and basic concepts
define, duplicate, list, memorize, repeat, state

Vanderbilt University Center for Teaching

FIGURE 7-3. Bloom's Taxonomy. ("Bloom's Taxonomy" by Center for Teaching Vanderbilt University is licensed under CC BY 2.0.)

determine, the answers. The mentor facilitates instead of trains. This will allow the employee to find their way, to try and sometimes fail, but learn through the process.

The mentor program should become a formal part of the practice, and a plan should be in place for each team member. Each department can identify a senior person, who is willing to assume additional responsibility, in assisting the new team member with learning how things are to be done. Recognizing the facilitator role, the mentor should be open and willing to ask questions, and to receive new ideas on how to improve. A formal program will have goals of the relationship, customer focus, time frame to accomplish with milestones (checkpoints), skills to be addressed, outputs from the effort, and the like.

Coaching is when an individual is available to offer technical advice. This advice may be highly technical, or even managerial, but is more of a 'how to,' rather than providing examples. The coach is typically the supervisor, or manager, of the team member. They function much the same as the athletic coach. For example, the coach is not in the game, but has trained the player how to do the job. When there is a time out, the coach is there to make suggestions, give further instructions, or congratulate for a job well done.

Here again, there is a need for a plan to be developed for everyone, since all team members have different skills. Referring to our athlete, it is expected to take up to 10,000 hours to achieve mastery in the chosen field of endeavor. That's equal to five years! Obviously, many tasks don't require that time frame, but the position just might.

MEASURING SUCCESS

A learning program is expensive, and therefore its return on investment, ROI, must be considered. The most cost-effective method to accomplish the objective must be explored.

As noted above, there are several goals that should be identified. When putting those goals together, it is necessary to keep in mind the expected outcome. Do you want a change in behavior, a change in the way things are done, improved patient satisfaction scores by what percentage, improved bottom line by dollar/ percent, or something else?

Ways then to measure effectiveness include:

- Observation – the trainer, or mentor, observes whether there has been improved performance.
- Social interaction – how staff interacts after training, or if the mentee shows more involvement with others.
- Skill assessments – test, demonstrations, and the like.

A key in this is the ongoing assessment. It is not enough to check out if change occurs with one observation, but instead to set up a schedule to follow up at specific, yet random, intervals. Very often staff will fall back to TW^{2}AI and not provide the improvement gain that is desired.

A part of the success should also lead to recognition for the employee. Is there a reward, such as a gift card, a dinner, or something similar? Is there a promotion in store for successful completion of the program? In developing a learning program, this aspect is also key when considering your ROI. Long lasting change in performance results will need to be measured.

Once a learning project is complete (e.g., you designed and implemented a program for a specific department, got an update on a mentoring project, etc.), it is a great time to follow the US Army and their After-Action Review, AAR. The individuals who put together the program, even the participants, can get together to and review the process and outcomes. They then can offer input on what can be done better, or recognize the items that went well. This concluding step to any learning effort is an excellent idea, and a great way to learn.

What does all this mean, and how does it translate to in the real world? A commitment to learning will:

- Retain employees. Cost of turnover is estimated at a minimum of 70% of annual earnings per position. This cost is in recruiting and loss of productivity. A check is not written, but resources are wasted, or not optimally utilized.
- Improve performance. A recent study in the journal, *Group & Organization Management*, reviewed 129 studies of training programs of physicians and clinicians who deliver healthcare, with more than 23,000 participants. "When training was implemented correctly, the result is improved outcomes across the board, both for patients and employees."[9]

- Improve patient outcomes. The same study found a reduction in mortality by 13%. How about that as a satisfaction survey result!
- Improve safety. Awareness of hazards in the office, double checking the right vs. left in procedures, etc. Effective policies, as well as corresponding training programs, achieve improved safety outcomes.
- Ensure compliance with required programs.

In most medical practices, the minimum education effort is undertaken, and typically limited to the required programs such as annual OSHA and HIPAA training. Little investment is made in the staff, which proves to be the most expensive asset. Maintenance fees are paid for software and hardware, and in some cases, these cost less than a single employee.

We know of one practice that includes 15 doctors, 10 locations, 250+ employees, and offers quarterly training. Each office is CLOSED the last Wednesday afternoon of the first three quarters. Their quarterly training breakdown is as follows:

- First quarter efforts at the required training, as well as offering optional training programs for all staff, all done on line. Staff remains at their work station, and tracking is done electronically.
- Second and third quarter staff assembles at a location for motivational and focused training on such things as customer service. Each function, such as receptionists from each office, get together to review procedures, seeking improvements in their operation.
- The last quarter involves a full day closure with a staff retreat. This includes education and networking opportunities, done at a resort. The staff is given the opportunity, at a reduced rate, to invite their families to enjoy the evening or weekend. Bus transportation is arranged from the offices as well.

One practice hired a trained teacher and taught her the issues of the medical practice. Her teaching and mentoring skills resulted in incredible feedback, reduced turnover, and improved patient outcomes.

Others have made a conscious effort by requiring monthly departmental meetings, with one component focused on an educational effort. This, often times, is general rather than practice specific. What it accomplishes is the attitude that learning is part of the culture of the practice.

Tuition reimbursement programs are a key in many practices. Here, the employee is reimbursed for college tuition on a course by course basis. If the results are a grade level or better, the payment is made with proof of the completion. Often, there is a requirement of continued employment for a period, such as one year after completion. If the employee leaves before that period, they pay back all, or a pro-rated portion, of the amount reimbursed. The course, or pathway, chosen typically relates to the employee's role or possible role, for example a medical assistant to registered nurse.

There is increased emphasis on the use of webinar, or other shared screen, options for training with either pre-purchased, internally developed, or live programs to reach staff in multiple locations.

REFERENCES

1. Senge PM. *The Fifth Discipline*. New York, NY: Penguin Random House; 2006
2. Yadav S. Argarwal V. Benefits and Barriers and Learning Organizations and its Five Discipline. *IOSR-Journal of Business and Management*. 2016;18:18-24 http://www.iosrjournals.org/iosr-jbm/papers/Vol18-issue12/Version-1/D1812011824.pdf
3. Pappas C. The Adult Learning Theory –Andragogy of Malcom Knowles. eLearning Industry. May 9, 2013; https://elearningindustry.com/the-adult-learning-theory-andragogy-of-malcolm-knowles. Accessed December 1. 2018.
4. Griggs, J. Generational Learning Styles (Generation X and Y) The Florida Institute of Technology. http://web2.fit.edu/ctle/documents/Course_Design/Generational%20Learning%20Styles%20Handout.pdf. Accessed December 1, 2018
5. Emotional Intelligence. Learning Theories. https://www.learning-theories.com/emotional-intelligence-goleman.html. Accessed December 1, 2018.
6. M. Libraries Publishing. http://open.lib.umn.edu/humanresourcemanagement/chapter/8-4-designing-a-training-program/. Accessed December 1. 2018.
7. Kirkpatrick, D. *Evaluating Training Programs*, 3rd ed. San Francisco, CA: Berrett-Koehler; 2006.
8. Vanderbilt University Center for Teaching. https://cft.vanderbilt.edu/guides-sub-pages/blooms-taxonomy/. December 1, 2018.
9. Shinkman R. Healthcare Team Training Cuts Patient Mortality , Study Finds, *FierceHealthcare*, March 13, 2018. Accessed December 1, 2018. https://www.fiercehealthcare.com/hospitals-health-systems/retraining-seen-as-way-to-cut-patient-mortality

SAMPLE ROLE PLAYS

At your employee meetings you can create from your own experience or use role play options that are available on the internet. Here is an example for two staff members to act out:

Role play – appointment schedule

Tom

> You need to telephone your doctor. You have an appointment on Tuesday the 3rd at 3:45 PM but you need to change it to Thursday the 5th at 3:00 PM. On Monday the 9th you are busy all day but Tuesday the 10th you have a free day.

> Telephone the doctor's clinic and speak to the receptionist. Make a new appointment

Role play – appointment schedule

Mary

> You are the receptionist at _____ (your practice) _____. You have no free appointments on Thursday the 5th as the doctor will be away that day. The next day the doctor is free is Monday the 9th.

> Answer the telephone and help the patient make a new appointment.

MENTORING AGREEMENT FORM

We are both voluntarily entering into this partnership. We wish this to be a rewarding experience, spending most of our time discussing developmental activities. We agree that . . .

1. The mentoring relationship will last for _____ months. This period will be evaluated every three to six months and will end by amicable agreement once we have achieved as much as possible.

2. We will meet at least once every _____ weeks. Meeting times, once agreed, should not be cancelled unless this is unavoidable. At the end of each meeting we will agree a date for the next meeting.

3. Each meeting will last a minimum of _____ minutes and a maximum of _____ minutes.

4. In between meetings we will contact each other by telephone/email no more than once every _____ weeks/days.

5. The aim of the partnership is to discuss and resolve the following issues:

6. We agree that the role of the mentor is to:

    _____

    _____

7. We agree that the role of the mentee is to:

    _____

    _____

8. We agree to keep the content of these meetings confidential.

9. The mentor agrees to be honest and provide constructive feedback to the mentee. The mentee agrees to be open to the feedback.

Date: _____

Mentor's signature: _____

Mentee's signature: _____

Date for Review: _____

Source: https://www.iop.org

CHARACTERISTICS OF A CONTINUOUSLY LEARNING HEALTH CARE SYSTEM

Use this table as a checklist for your learning system:

TABLE: Characteristics of a Continuously Learning Health Care System

Science and Informatics

- **Real-time access to knowledge**—A learning health care system continuously and reliably captures, curates, and delivers the best available evidence to guide, support, tailor, and improve clinical decision making and care safety and quality.

- **Digital capture of the care experience**—A learning health care system captures the care experience on digital platforms for real-time generation and application of knowledge for care improvement.

Patient-Clinician Relationships

- **Engaged, empowered patients**—A learning health care system is anchored on patient needs and perspectives and promotes the inclusion of patients, families, and other caregivers as vital members of the continuously learning care team.

Incentives

- **Incentives aligned for value**—In a learning health care system, incentives are actively aligned to encourage continuous improvement, identify and reduce waste, and reward high-value care.

- **Full transparency**—A learning health care system systematically monitors the safety, quality, processes, prices, costs, and outcomes of care, and makes information available for care improvement and informed choices and decision making by clinicians, patients, and their families.

Culture

- **Leadership-instilled culture of learning**—A learning health care system is stewarded by leadership committed to a culture of teamwork, collaboration, and adaptability in support of continuous learning as a core aim.

- **Supportive system competencies**—In a learning health care system, complex care operations and processes are constantly refined through ongoing team training and skill building, systems analysis and information development, and creation of the feedback loops for continuous learning and system improvement.

Source: http://www.nationalacademies.org/hmd/Reports/2012/Best-Care-at-Lower-Cost-The-Path-to-Continuously-Learning-Health-Care-in-America/Table.aspx

Chapter 8

Healthcare Practice Finances: RCM (Revenue Cycle Management) and Patient Responsibility

Most practices today do an adequate job managing revenue cycle issues in the fee-for-service world. We will review the main items briefly, but the key is how, and what, is done with the value-based and alternative payment model options today. Additionally, it is important to identify what it costs, and how you manage these costs of providing care. We will discuss this in greater detail.

REVENUE CYCLE BASICS

The top line, collections for services provided, can be complex to manage. Yet, with adequate staff, training, and a solid practice management software, this has become more routine for most practices. The basic cycle is noted in Figure 8-1.

The cycle starts with the initial contact from the patient. It is necessary to gather all demographic and insurance information to ensure accurate set up of the account, and a thorough check for valid insurance coverage. This can occur via phone, or internet connection. If done through the internet, the patient should complete all necessary business and clinical forms. These should be reviewed to eliminate asking the same question more than once, as asking the same question multiple times can frustrate a patient. In addition, the patient should be directed to review the financial policy, which indicates their responsibility and the tasks to be done by the practice on their behalf.

The financial policy is a simple, but complete, statement outlining patient responsibility. It is important that the patient review, and sign, this document. This ensures their understanding of things like co-pay, deductible, and past due balance management issues and collection point policies, as well as removes stress from front desk staff when the patient checks in or checks out. Content of the policy should include, at a minimum, the following items:

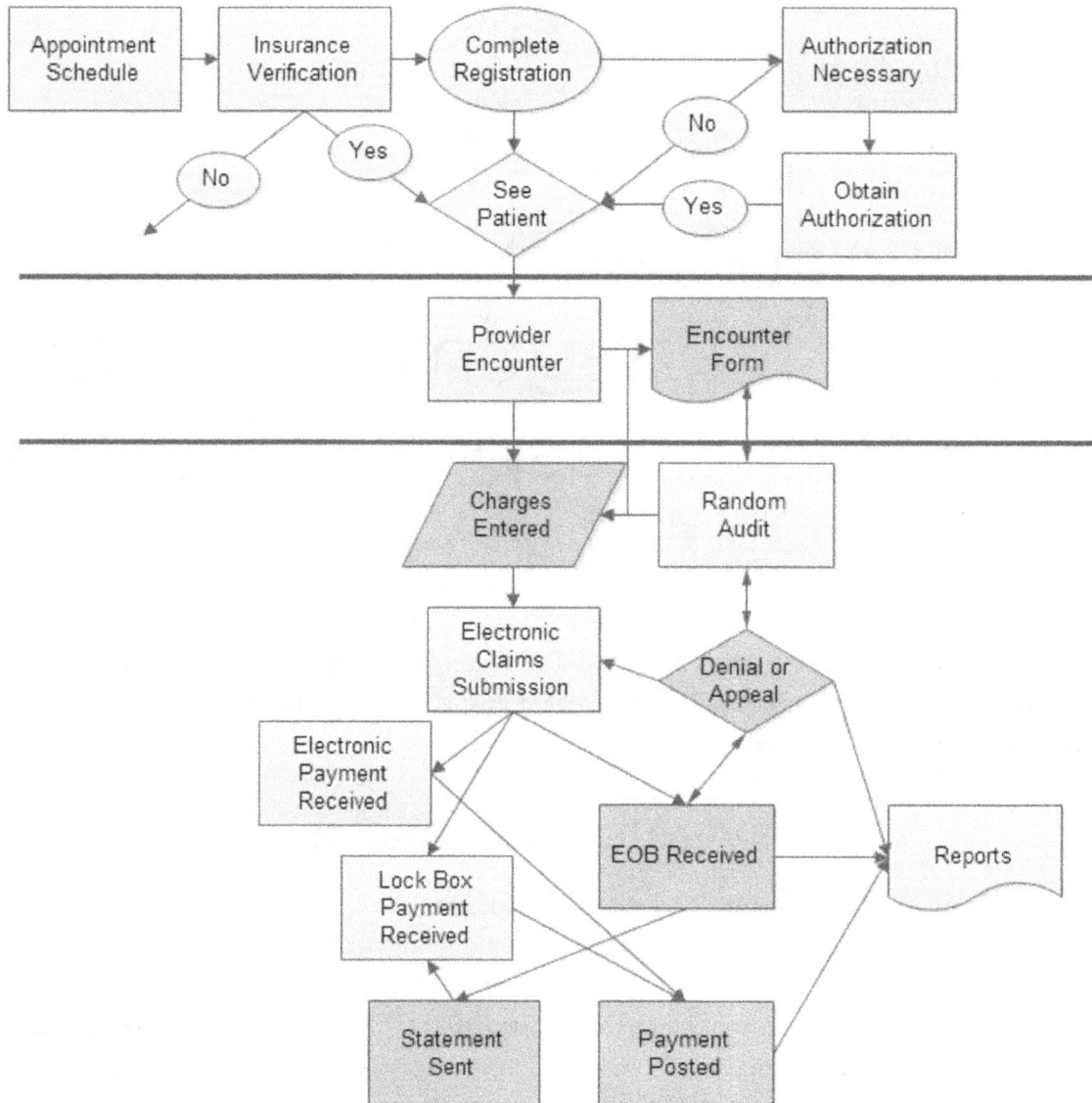

FIGURE 8-1. Basic Revenue Cycle

- Introduction – what is in this policy?
- Patient is responsible for what they owe
- When payments are expected
- Fees for late payments; discount options
- If they don't pay, what could happen
- Allow for discounts for cash payments
- Consider charging for sending statements (incentive to pay on time, discounts)
- Signature

In addition to this, a collection policy should be developed by practice leadership that spells out, in detail, the 'how to,' and 'what is to be done,' in managing the entire revenue cycle. For example, leadership agrees that all payments must be made prior to any service provided, or the patient will be asked to re-schedule. This eliminates questions and issues faced often by the front desk staff. There may be some exceptions allowed, such as obvious need for care to avoid liability, or if the patient forgot their wallet but have paid each time for the last 10 visits (instead of only two). Other items include what, how much, when, and how to turn a patient to a collection agency. Define a delinquent account (typically two statements past due). How do you handle low payments from insurance carriers? How do you handle multiple family members? Questions like these must be acknowledged. This policy should be consistent and built on the financial policy. Thinking this through and agreeing on the guidelines will save time and reduce stress.

There should be key performance indicators, KPI, which are established as goals for the revenue cycle results. These include, but are not limited to:

- Days in accounts receivable – the ratio of average daily charges (total charges per day over the last 180 days) divided into the total accounts receivable. This should be tracked monthly and trend monitored. The KPI would be less than 30 days, depending upon specialty, case and payer mix.
- Net collectable percentage – the ratio of collectable amounts (charges minus contractual rates paid) divided by actual amounts collected. KPI is 95% or better.
- Percentage of accounts over 120 days – in the aged trial balance, the amount of dollars in 120 days, or older 'buckets,' should be no more than a KPI of 10%. This should be monitored for the amount written off with no arbitrary write offs allowed. All write offs should be defined in the collection policy.

After covering the basics, we must further the deep dive by asking the next question. What needs to be done to meet today's real revenue cycle challenges? As mentioned previously, this is the time to incorporate a learning organization. There is so much information in the market, and so many changes occurring in today's medical practice reimbursement process, that it is impossible to rest on the one, or two things, that are done well. Helping the staff to learn the principles, and what's behind these changes, will encourage them to seek ways to improve the overall revenue cycle management needs.

As the move continues to value-based, there will be alternative payment models, APM, to consider. See Figure 8-2.

The traditional fee-for-service, FFS, model, considered frequently as pay-for-volume rather than outcomes, is on the left. Insurance carriers have paid for this based on submission of a procedure code, CPT®, and a diagnosis code, now ICD-10. The way that payers have chosen to address this is via prior authorization based upon some level of evidence

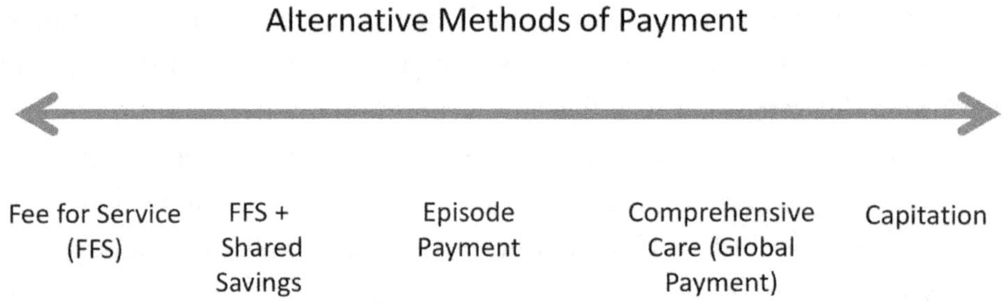

Alternative Methods of Payment

| Fee for Service (FFS) | FFS + Shared Savings | Episode Payment | Comprehensive Care (Global Payment) | Capitation |

FIGURE 8-2. Payment Continuum

to justify either level of code in the case of visits or procedures deemed either necessary or unnecessary per their guidelines. This has added frustration, and cost, to the medical practice.

There are many hybrid models on the market today, starting with the FFS and shared savings. Payers have their formulas, which we will not address here. Instead, understand that there are incentive programs, even within the FFS world.

More likely methods include episodic and global payments. There are many definitions for these methods, but for our purposes let's use the following. The episodic is payment per episode. This method is like a surgical procedure, with defined services included for a period related to the primary diagnosis. This expands the concept to medical services and may include chronic treatments for a designated amount of time. Typically, these are paid to one provider rather than several. DRG paid to hospital, and three months of diabetic care paid to an endocrinologist, are examples of this.

Comprehensive payments include all services provided for a diagnosis. An example of the payee would be an ACO. Funds paid would be distributed to all providers involved, such as hospital, imaging center, physician(s), and the like. The payer has negotiated a contract for all services with the ACO, and it is up to the ACO to distribute the funds per their agreements.

Capitation has been around for several years, and is basically a per member, per month method. The payer agrees to pay a provider (physician, hospital, or ACO) an agreed upon amount per subscriber, per month, regardless of what services are provided, if any, to the patient during that month.

These later payment models shift the risk of care provided from the payer to the provider, to whatever extent all parties agree to accept the terms of the agreement. We will review more on this later.

The big issue, in this section, is how to manage these different payment methods within the existing software system(s) in the office. Here are some questions for you to address in your revenue cycle process:

- High deductible health plans, HDHP, require significant dollars directly from the patient.

– Issues surround whether a deposit or advance is required, even for routine visits as well as procedures.

– How do you handle patients who do not pay at each visit?

• What negotiation should occur with payers who want to utilize one of the 'risks' based or incentive methods or payment?

– What is your cost?

– What is your target margin?

– What dollar amount or "hassle factor" (pre-authorization, care plan compliance) are you willing to accept or walk away from?

– What is the termination clause?

– What terms relate to payment level changes?

• In a comprehensive care model who will you be negotiating with and what terms are acceptable?

• In managing claims do you want to continue to post each service as a charge?

– When do you adjust charges that are paid under a 'bulk' method, such as episodic or capitation?

– What options are there to determine productivity of each provider?

• The big one – how to handle compensation for each service provided?

– Primary provider?

– Each provider for each service?

There are no simple answers to any of these questions. Traditional guidance suggests still tracking productivity, including who does what, what services are provided within a defined care plan to ensure evidence-based care is provided, if available resources are utilized, if patients are managed in an efficient manner. Be sure to train staff about these new options and get their involvement in the 'how to' best model, to ensure adequate reporting and monitoring occurs for quality, as well as financial results.

COST MANAGEMENT

A very simple question to ask is, "how much does it cost to see a patient?" Qualify that with an established 99213 level of care patient. Typically, when asked, most do not have an answer to this question. This is both shocking, and scary, when we consider the above discussion on different reimbursement methods. It is impossible to manage the practice without knowing the cost of doing business.

Let's look at a simple one doctor primary care practice, as an example. Table 8-1 gives us a good picture:

TABLE 8-1. Typical Financial Statement, Solo Primary Care Practice

Model Financial Statement			
	Annual	**% Income**	**Per Visit**
All Sources Income	$579,794	100.00%	$92.77
Expenses			
Bank charge	$1,011	0.17%	$0.16
Billing service	$16,368	2.82%	$2.62
Communication	$6,299	1.09%	$1.01
Contributions	$183	0.03%	$0.03
Depreciation	$8,410	1.45%	$1.35
Dues & Sub	$2,893	0.50%	$0.46
Ins - Bus & Mal	$12,400	2.14%	$1.98
Ins - Employee	$16,255	2.80%	$2.60
Legal & Acct	$6,131	1.06%	$0.98
Marketing	$9,055	1.56%	$1.45
Med supplies	$33,618	5.80%	$5.38
Ofc exp	$17,912	3.09%	$2.87
Payroll	$136,094	23.47%	$21.78
Payroll tax	$10,581	1.82%	$1.69
Rent	$55,491	9.57%	$8.88
Rep & Maint	$1,123	0.19%	$0.18
Taxes	$1,337	0.23%	$0.21
Training	$53	0.01%	$0.01
Total Expenses	$335,214	57.82%	$53.63
Net income	$244,580	42.18%	$39.13

The typical way to look at this is to consider the total income, $579,794, as a barometer of how well things are doing. This figure is used to determine the overhead percentage, here 57.82%. The % income column then reveals the percentage associated with each line item of expense. There may be other columns reflecting this year to last year, this year's actual to budget, or the data being presented on a month to month basis. Discussion, and analysis, then follows this presentation. One observation could be that overhead is too high, there is a need to cut, and since that the biggest line item is employee expense, let's cut employees. The four employees are paid an average of $34,000, or $16.36 per hour. Depending upon your market, this should be representative and therefore, not an issue. The strategy of first cutting overtime is popular. But what results have followed? Overtime is controlled for a month or two, and then creeps back up!

Instead, look at the column on the right. This begins to answer the question of total cost to see one patient. Here we have grouped all patient visits (new, established, hospital, etc.) in to the equation. This may not be totally accurate but gives us a good place start. First, the revenue per visit is noted at $92.77, which is higher than what Medicare pays for a 99213 (~$70+). The $53.63 cost per visit does not includes the physician. The balance is what is taken home, so the profit per visit it $39.13, a 42% margin. These are not bad results, even with a greater than 50% overhead figure. If four patients are seen per hour, that's an hourly equivalent of $160 per hour.

With this in mind, let's then further analyze by breaking down the patient count, and allocation of expense to new patients and hospital patients. If procedures are involved, further detail is necessary and can be created. Instead of per visit, it is possible to look at variation, such as per total relative value unit, RVU, or work RVU. This may be more effective since current FFS models for reimbursement, and many for compensation, are built on the RVU model.

This can be taken one step further in relation to the value-based payment reimbursement options. Per visit, or per RVU, may not be the best alternative. Instead, there is an option referred to as time driven activity-based cost, TDABC. This requires a little more work, but in the long run will address all issues surrounding what services are provided, and their related costs.

The definition of TDABC starts with a basic understanding "Activity-based costing (ABC) is a costing methodology that identifies activities in an organization and assigns the cost of each activity with resources to all products and services according to the actual consumption by each."[1] (The TD portion simply adds time as a key use of resources.) This is critical in health care, since time is a major factor in all activities. To be successful in developing a TDABC model, there are two critical items. The first is to understand the resources necessary to address the demand. The second is to understand the time.

Recall the discussion on time, value add, non-value add, and business value add services provided per patient visit. We looked at an average established patient visit in a primary care practice. Let's apply this model with the details noted in Table 8-2. The one physician has four full time employees, a patient panel of 2, 500, and sees 6,250 visits per year, for an average of 26 per day for the 240 days the office is open. This translates to 368,640 minutes worked per employee, which is capacity. This includes the 1,920 hours worked for the 240 days, minus 20% for administration time, personal time, training time, etc. The employees are productive 6,144 minutes per year. This equates then to 59 minutes per visit. This time can then be looked at as value, non-value, and business value time.

TABLE 8-2. TDABC worksheet

Primary Care	
One Physician	
Four full time employees	
Patient Panel	2,500
Annual Patient Visits	6,250
Patients seen per day (240 days)	26
Paid hours (2,080*4)	8,320
Work hours (240 days/year)	7,680
Net work hours (-20%)	6,144
Net minutes worked (capacity)	368,640
Hours per visit	0.98
Minutes per visit	58.98
Employee Cost per minute	$0.44
Total cost per minute	$0.91
Patients seen per day	26
Increase one	27
Total patients seen	6,490
Hours per visit	0.95
Minutes per visit	56.8
Total time gained per visit	2.18

What is the cost per minute, and how does that help better manage finances in the new reimbursement world? Combine the value stream map and the TDABC model and see if we can make sense out of all of this.

We see in Table 8-2 that the employee cost per minute is $.44, total cost $.91. Employee costs include payroll, payroll taxes, employee insurance, and training. Since we are concerned with time, we will look only at employee costs. As the second aspect of our definition notes there could, and should be, additional analysis on the other resources, and their related line item costs to fully understand all resources that go into the activity being measured. Or, you could run the same approach considering all costs.

In Table 8-3, we find some very interesting data. First, the business value cost per visit is $3.52, value add $11.00, and non-value add $11.44, for a total employee cost of $25.96 per 59-minute visit (total staff time available and applied to each visit). Recognize the non-value time is wasted; we have calculated a cost related to waste. This is critical to our understanding of both the Lean concepts, as well as the cost of doing business. In this example, we cut four minutes of non-value add time which reduced the cost per visit. This frees up staff time to apply to other activities.

TABLE 8-3. Value vs. Other Time and Costs

Activity	Business Value	Value	Non Value	Total	Employee Per Visit Cost	New	Revised Cost
Check-in	4			4	$1.76	4	$1.76
Reception			17	17	$7.48	15	$6.60
Triage		8		8	$3.52	8	$3.52
Wait			4	4	$1.76	3	$1.32
Provider		12		12	$5.28	12	$5.28
Wait			3	3	$1.32	2	$0.88
Post		5		5	$2.20	5	$2.20
Wait			2	2	$0.88	2	$0.88
Check- out	4			4	$1.76	4	$1.76
Total	8	25	26	59	$25.96	55	$24.20
	$3.52	$11.00	$11.44	$25.96		Saved 4 minutes of non-value add	
PCE	42.37%						
New PCE	45.45%						

By looking at the value-add time provided in each step, we discovered some duplication of activities. This did not result in a direct savings of value-add time, but did reduce the wait time in two steps, one minute each. This helped reduce the wait time in the reception area by two minutes. This four-minute savings reduced total time by four minutes, and a cost reduction of $1.76 per visit.

We have added a calculation at the bottom of Table 8-3 called the PCE. PCE is process cycle efficiency. This tracks how much time of the actual visit produces value add time. Our initial PCE was 42.37%, and after a few adjustments, we improved to 45.45%. There is no standard intended here. Instead, this is simply an introduction to another metric that could be used to measure efficiency.

Remember, this example does not include the cost saving that could occur from other resources such as table paper, tongue depressors, and other basic items. If seeing one more patient at 99213 Medicare rates netted about $18,000 per year, there would be some increased costs in supplies. But these increased costs are considered minimal, when acknowledging the world of FFS.

This entire change resulted in improved patient satisfaction scores, which improved the value-based payment reimbursement figures. Plus, reducing patient cycle time in non-value add areas improved the time available for staff to complete additional tasks, allowing them to finish on time, or early. This then translates into an overtime cost savings, or employee satisfaction improvement.

Using the process map tool, and the TDABC model, the practice has seen significant benefit in the many areas noted.

RETURN ON INVESTMENT

The return on investment calculation is easy, necessary, and not always followed up on once calculated. Due diligence is exercised in making an investment decision but is not always reviewed periodically to ensure that the projections were correct, or explore what went wrong. The formula is very simple:

$$ROI = (Net\ profit/cost\ of\ investment)\ x\ 100$$

A $1,000 investment with a profit of $200 yields a return of 20% for that period. This can be measured over months, or years, depending upon what the investment involves.

In making this calculation, it is necessary to clearly understand what the expenses are to operate and/or manage the investment. It is necessary to understand all sources of income, and then determine the net profit for the defined period. The tricky part is that an ROI calculation is flexible, a benefit, but it can also be manipulated in many ways at both the revenue, and expense, level.

We would encourage the practice to make its own ROI calculation, and not rely on a vendor. This is important since the practice has knowledge of its own expenses, sources of revenue, and can control all aspects at the initial phase. The practice can then accurately compare the projections to the actual results during the follow up.

The ROI is not only beneficial when considering the purchase of capital equipment. It is useful when considering a new program. For example, if the practice is moving ahead in a value-based purchasing program, there are at least two additional expenditures that are required. The first is increased, or improved, analytics. This may require additional software, or modification of current software. It may also require hiring a data analyst. Both are capital, and personnel, consideration. Further, typically the practice will need to hire, or secure the services of, a care manager or service. This, again, may require upgrades to software and additional staff. What is the expected cost/benefit or ROI for this new program? The answer here is not important, but it is important to consider the question.

COMPENSATION

This is a difficult subject, and often leads to decisions to split the group or join with another group, or healthcare system. So often we have seen groups attempt to manipulate the compensation formula to be fair to all. When there are mixed specialties, it is difficult to do so.

Typical options for compensation are 100% production, receipts / RVU/ some related model, 100% salary, or a combination with a portion equal and the balance based on production or some other key factor. The interesting point is when the focus is 100% production for a practice of 12 physicians, you end up with 12 different cultures. This creates issues as we look to the future with value-based payment changes from FFS, and the goal of population health management. How does one address the goal of volume, incentive to increase production, combined with the concept of bringing value, and reducing waste? Stark laws have reduced some of the excess testing incentive, with the restrictions on compensation for imaging and other testing. However, malpractice cases encourage more testing, and those concerned about this are incentivized to do more testing. This is somewhat of a side issue but is important when considering the best model for compensation.

Recent literature has pointed out that the successful groups are those with salary models, rather than production models. Larger clinics have chosen the salaried approach, which is paying a fair salary for the work required by the physician. But this may not be the best alternative for a small to mid-size group.

The compromise of a portion of compensation equal, combined with a portion based on production, seems to work well. This may be a good solution for those 100% productivity groups that are facing a market driven by value-based payment models. The transition period with this compromise will help all understand the issues better and help work toward a stable model.

As an administrator, the goal has been to provide data and stay away from direct discussions. One physician that I have had the privilege to work with made the most valid comment related to compensation. Consider this: when the board gets together for the annual compensation discussion, if everyone leaves a little disappointed, the result is positive. If one or a few leave happy, others won't, and there will be issues in the future.

GUIDELINES VS. PATHWAYS

This may seem to be a strange place to include a discussion on the clinical aspects of treating a patient, but it is not. Value-based payments will be based upon outcomes, and compliance with treatment plans. Let's define a couple key terms. First, a guideline is an evidence-based approach to providing care to the patient. This evidence emerges from various recognized sources, such as specialty society published findings of key research studies, or the government. Second, the pathway is the standardization of the care process.

Evidence-based information indicates which procedures, diagnostic test, medications, and treatment regimens have worked for patients who present with a disease state. There may be two, or three, acceptable approaches that can be presented to the patient, or decided upon by the physician. It is best if a committee recommends, or the group decides and accepts the best option(s) and encourages care decisions based upon what the group has determined. It is important to note that care must be exercised when accepting the research results based upon sponsorship of the study, as the results could be swayed by the investor.

Pathways take the three options and develops the best mechanism to deliver each in the most efficient fashion possible. A pathway will include not only the direct medical treatment, but the entire supporting structure to achieve the best possible outcome in the most efficient manner possible.

Let's return to the basics of finance. We reviewed cost from a global and practice level. One of the big moves today is transparency. This means that consumers – employers and individuals – are concerned about cost of care. When reviewing the web, you see scholarly articles related to the need to meet public demands, and awareness of the cost of care. The increase in high deductible health plans, HDHP, and uninsured patients creates more need of awareness to what is happening in your market. Here's a comment from the Blue Cross Blue Shield of Michigan web site:

> "You have choices when it comes to care
>
> You compare costs for plane tickets, TVs and even new laptops. So why not do the same for your health care?
>
> If you're a Blue Cross member with a qualifying plan, you can log in to get estimates for services ranging from routine tests to complex surgeries. Then choose the option that's right for you and your wallet."[2]

It will become more critical to manage your pricing of services. Pricing of these services cannot be based solely on what the others are charging, or what payers are offering. They must be based upon the cost of providing care.

Beyond the revenue and cost side, there is also the need to provide value to the patient. A cost benefit equation not only considers the out lay of dollars, but what the return on the investment yields.

What we have found includes the following scenarios:

- Repeating the content of the financial statement and what it means.
  - Making the format simple
  - Keeping the format, the same or similar
  - Pointing out the key performance indicators, KPI
  - Offering comparison from year-to-year, budget to actual, or benchmark from other practices such as through MGMA data solutions, or from professional societies
- The CFO or CPA who is great with generating numbers and reports but offer no analysis.
  - Time for training (see previous chapter) or personnel change
- Non-integrated electronic medical record and practice management system.
  - Combine the data bases to get consistent reporting materials
  - Clinical outcomes must relate to financial income and cost
- Not knowing what reports are available, and valuable.
  - Practice management systems provide a denial report, and so does the clearinghouse with different data.
- Getting too much information, and not being able to sort what makes the most sense.
- Determining the best approach to cost analysis by visit, service line, RVU, and again, even the importance of this exercise itself.
- Lack of knowledge or resources to benchmark key performance indicators in areas of finance, compensation, production, or efficiency management.

REFERENCES

1. Wikipedia: https://en.wikipedia.org/wiki/Activity-based_costing). Accessed December 1, 2018
2. Blue Cross, Blue Shield of Michigan. "You Have Choices When it Comes to Care," https://www.bcbsm.com/understand-cost/index.html. Accessed December 1, 2018

REVENUE CYCLE MANAGEMENT TASK LIST

Central Telephone

Appointment schedule
- Matrix/schema per office and/or provider
- Schedule patient for appropriate time
- Demographic information
- Insurance information

Reminder call
- 24 – 48 hours prior to appointment call to remind, seek confirmation
  - If automated get report and review prior to leaving for day
- Identify those with balances and indicate that amount is to be paid at the visit
  - Personal call for those with balances due

Received calls (all staff)
- Answer with four part greeting
  - Time of day, e.g., good morning
  - Name of practice
  - Your name
  - Query – "how may I help you"
- Transfer call
  - Ask permission
  - Give reason why
  - Give phone number/extension
  - Indicate who will be answering the phone
- Place on hold
  - Ask permission
  - Pick up and say thank you
  - Extend greeting
  - Respond to request

Clinic locations

Front desk
- Receive patient, not just greet
  - Verify name
  - Verify house number, not total address
  - Verify last four of phone number, not total phone number

- Notify triage that patient has arrived
- Indicate where patient can sit
- Maintain clean reception area at all times

Check in/out
- Collect co-pay and deductible amounts due (major item starting January 1 each year with deductible amounts due especially from Medicare patients) Only collect up to allowable amount.
- Schedule for follow up visit and/or outside diagnostic or treatments as necessary

Coding Department

Coding
- Physicians determine the level of code and note in the system
- Staff will audit random documentation to ensure that proper coding levels are billed
- Staff will inform physicians of the findings of the audit as well as any changes in coding that are identified with the annual CPT publication, local carrier determination, LCD, and the correct coding initiative, CCI

Billing department

Claims processing
- Correct data entry will allow for the generation of the claim which should be done daily

Claims scrub report
- Initial claims processed through the clearinghouse will result in a report of those claims that are not clean
- These claims should be reviewed immediately and prepared for resubmission
- Data from this process should be gathered and prepared for necessary education and/or re-training of the appropriate staff

EOB processing
- Payments posted daily
- Denials are noted on appropriate task list and forwarded for processing
- Flag for secondary submissions for those claims not automatically filed, claims submitted daily

Denial management
- Check the task list for activity
- Process daily ALL denials and resubmit claims as appropriate
- If an appeal is determined necessary, gather the data and submit to carrier for review

COST CALCULATION TEMPLATES

Cost to see a patient*
$$\frac{\text{Total expense}}{\text{Total visits}} = \text{Cost per visit}$$
* select time period, e.g, month, year for both measures
* select metric, e.g., wRVU, tRVU instead of visits

Cost to provide a service*
$$\frac{\text{Identified function/department}}{\text{Total contacts}} = \text{Cost per contact}$$
* select function, e.g., triage, check in
* select department, e.g., imaging, lab

Takt Time
Wages per hour/60 = cost per minute
$$\frac{\text{Tme associated with function}}{\text{Cost per minute}} = \text{Labor cost to do function}$$
$$\frac{\text{Resource cost for function}}{\text{Cost per contact}} = \text{Resource cost to do function}$$
* select function, e.g., triage, check in
* select department, e.g., imaging, lab

Chapter 9

Benefits of Technology in Clinical Operations

What comes to mind when you hear the word, technology? Computers, digital, Smart phones, AI? When we look at the official definition, we find something broader. Technology "is the collection of techniques, skills, methods, and processes used in the production of goods or services or in the accomplishment of objectives." Further, technology can be knowledge of the above, "or it can be embedded in machines."[1] Technology incorporates everything from fire, the wheel, the printing press, the telephone, and even the internet.

In today's medical practice, we think that technology will help make us more efficient. Yet, in many cases, that result is unseen. So much technology has been developed that it is difficult to keep up with everything. There is Moore's law, which predicts that the cost of computing will be cut in half. Therefore, why get involved now, when instead you can wait for tomorrow, since it will only be better? Over the past decade, the medical practice has been encouraged by regulations and incentives to implement the EMR. Prior to this, the computer had become indispensable for billing and overall practice management. Today, we must explore technology and move into the realm of improved clinical management of patients.

At the end of each calendar year, experts identify what technology, new and expanded, will be popular for the next year. Here is a sample of what was noted at a recent year end:

- Three-D printing and images for medical education
- Wearables, "insideables"
- Genome sequencing
- IoT – Internet of Things
- Bio-electronics
- Robotics
- Telemedicine
- Blockchain
- AI - Artificial intelligence
- Reality – virtual, augmented, and actual

This is not intended to be a complete, up-to-date list. And applications for the medical office, medical device, and pharmaceutical industry are unknown at this point.

Has technology made the office more efficient, more patient friendly, and helped identify value savings, in time and costs? Or, has it become a bigger burden to, what is already, a complex environment? Jonathan Gruber, one of the architects of the ACA, has noted that "Computers make things better and cheaper. In health care, new technology makes things better, but more expensive."[2] Digital technology is here to stay, but in this chapter, we will explore how to manage it, and take advantage of what it has to offer.

EMR OR EHR

If we look at the integration of the EMR/EHR into the practice, the basic outcome is that there is more work, more time required, less focus on the patient, for a typically unknown benefit. Many of the issues in implementation are found in the changes of payment models with PQRI(S), APM, MIPS, and many more acronyms. Many feel that the EMR was forced upon the practice, and that there has been little planning related to the implementation. Many practices have assumed that it would work with a little technical training on how to use the tool. This has resulted in longer patient visits, poor patient contact, and an increased cost of care.

A recent article in the *Harvard Business Review* addressed IT transformation in health care. As we have noted previously, it is good to see how other industries function when compared to healthcare. Figure 9-1 is most revealing about productivity:[3]

Despite the overall growth in employment in healthcare, one of the most growth-oriented areas in the US economy, overall gains in productivity, lag most all other industries. The article sites that two key areas – senior leadership and clinicians – should place a greater emphasis on the use of IT in providing care and developing data to ensure appropriate outcomes. The simple addition of the EMR/EHR has added to the stress, leading to the burnout, noted earlier.

Instead of throwing technology into the existing care process, it would be beneficial to understand what the existing system entails. A practice with five providers has five different approaches to the use of the tool. The use of Lean management tools, such as a process map, could have save a lot of pain. This would mean looking at how things are done in each of the five practices prior to EHR implementation (although, it may now be too late). Stop now and create a process map for each provider. See what road blocks exist, and what things work well. Talk it over, and work with the support staff to find, and implement, new and more efficient ways to proceed.

Here are some key points on overall technology that a healthcare practice should consider:

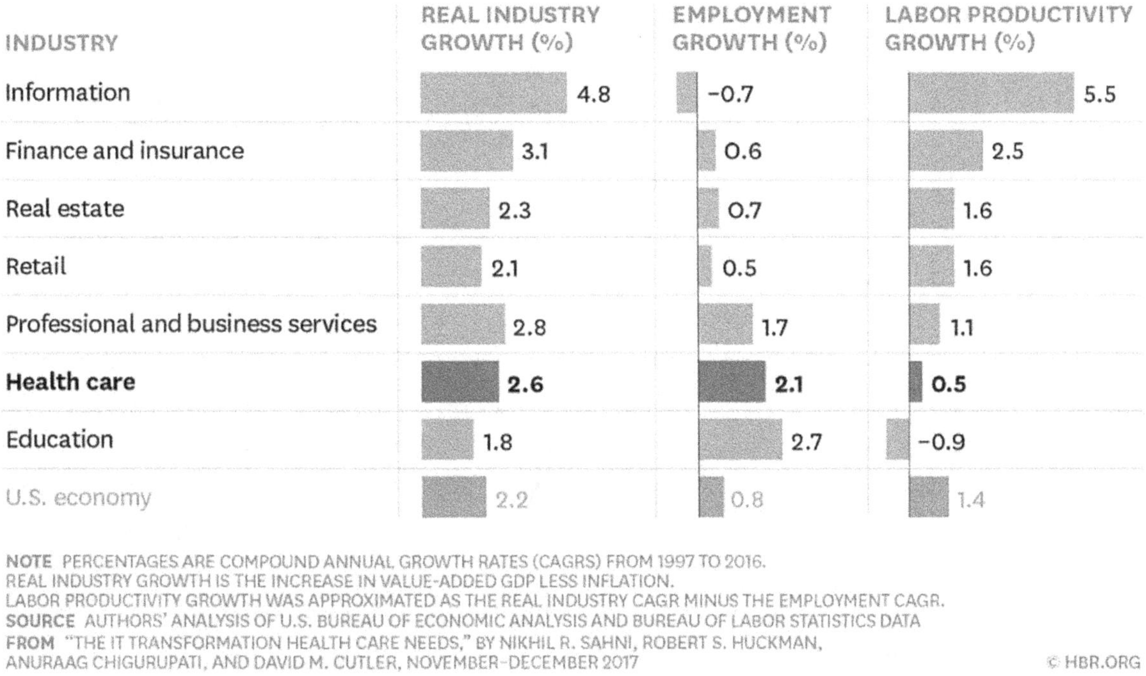

INDUSTRY	REAL INDUSTRY GROWTH (%)	EMPLOYMENT GROWTH (%)	LABOR PRODUCTIVITY GROWTH (%)
Information	4.8	-0.7	5.5
Finance and insurance	3.1	0.6	2.5
Real estate	2.3	0.7	1.6
Retail	2.1	0.5	1.6
Professional and business services	2.8	1.7	1.1
Health care	**2.6**	**2.1**	**0.5**
Education	1.8	2.7	-0.9
U.S. economy	2.2	0.8	1.4

NOTE PERCENTAGES ARE COMPOUND ANNUAL GROWTH RATES (CAGRS) FROM 1997 TO 2016.
REAL INDUSTRY GROWTH IS THE INCREASE IN VALUE-ADDED GDP LESS INFLATION.
LABOR PRODUCTIVITY GROWTH WAS APPROXIMATED AS THE REAL INDUSTRY CAGR MINUS THE EMPLOYMENT CAGR.
SOURCE AUTHORS' ANALYSIS OF U.S. BUREAU OF ECONOMIC ANALYSIS AND BUREAU OF LABOR STATISTICS DATA
FROM "THE IT TRANSFORMATION HEALTH CARE NEEDS," BY NIKHIL R. SAHNI, ROBERT S. HUCKMAN,
ANURAAG CHIGURUPATI, AND DAVID M. CUTLER, NOVEMBER–DECEMBER 2017   © HBR.ORG

https://hbr.org/2017/11/the-it-transformation-health-care-needs

FIGURE 9-1. Productivity in Various Industries

- Cloud – rather than investing in infrastructure, use of the cloud provides elasticity; allowing for use, and paying only for what you need. This is a key in managing disasters that occur too often. In addition, there is improved access to key practice documents. It is also a less expensive option for storage and reliability.
- IoT – the internet of Things — giving access to devices from other practices and to the patient and their wearable devices.
- Big data – there is more information available now more than ever, but the question is how to access it. It is indicated that in the future, up to 25% of the patients EMR will contain data directly from the patient.
- Cybersecurity – this is the scary part. The many stories of hacking and ransom demands cause many sleepless nights.
- Blockchain – is "an open, distributed ledger that can record transactions between two parties efficiently and in a verifiable and permanent way."[4] In theory, this is a secure, trusted, and shared document path. Once written, the data can be modified or edited, but the original cannot be changed. Applications include managing supply chain with vendors and pharma, recruitment of patients for clinical trials, and improved security and interoperability.

- Artificial Intelligence – Stephen Hawking is afraid of this and has called this," the worst event in the history of civilization unless society finds a way to control its development."[5] Others feel that this concept will augment people and become a key tool for success in areas of diagnosis and treatment of patients, such as IBM's Watson.
- Precision Medicine. The use of genetic information to create customized, improved use of biologics.

A big question for each practice is what to do in the future. Do you need more digital applications, or is what you are doing adequate? Can you join with others (in some fashion, to be determined) to benefit from advances, and focus only on the business side, or focus only on the clinical side?

From a clinical perspective you could consider three approaches:

1. Basic, low cost with benefit to many – past efforts like low-cost antibiotics, simple casts, and the like. Typically, low cost, but the key is who and how many will receive a benefit.
2. Benefits substantial for a few patients, and the application or demand for those technologies in your practice.
3. Benefit few, early technology, not necessarily proven, but has potential. These are typically very expensive, and you must consider if you want to be an early adapter, or a follower.[6]

When we look at this the cost benefit, the simple equation looks at efficiency + benefit over cost. Consider this from both a global, as well as local (your practice), perspective. The global question is well beyond the scope of this book, but still must be in the minds of the individuals who will consider application of the new technology in their local practice.

One of the goals in this book is to encourage the reader to look at their role in the greater scheme of things, e.g., population management. Technology with big data, patient tracking, observation through telemedicine, and the like will certainly help in dealing with access to care, as well as development and implementation of wellness programs.

Eric Topol in his book *The Creative Destruction of Medicine*, raises the counter argument.[7] Topol is a cardiologist amd a geneticist and looks at the technological changes as helping define care at the individual level instead of at the population level. A conundrum, but at the same time something that requires a dual focus in the decision-making process of the practice.

The incidents of cyber breaches continue to increase. For the individual practice, it is important to look at three aspects of protection:

- Detection – what tools, steps, devices are in place to assist with detection of a breach. We hear many stories about the detection of a breach occurring several weeks or even months before it is detected.

- Protection – an area that is always in focus. Backup systems, the cloud, and external options work well. Firewalls must be built in. But it always seems that the hackers are one step ahead of the protectors. There are conferences where convicted, and/or expert hackers, get together to show their skills and offer to vendors new and better ways to include protection in their systems.

- Response – this is a weak area that needs to be seriously considered in system planning, and certainly when hacked. The FBI may be very interested in a hack. You may have local experts who have experience. For example, consider if your practice is hacked and there is a ransom attached for $2M. Do you give in, do you negotiate, or do you risk the public disclosure of the HIPAA violation, causing additional expense as well as impacting your reputation? How serious is the threat and the cost/benefit of dealing with it?

A recent article from McKinsey & Company identifies seven building blocks for the management of digital risk.[8] These blocks are:

1. Data management – this includes a focus on decision making and governance, as well as the operation of your system. Infrastructure is always a key in all aspects of decision making.

2. Process and work flow automation – as mentioned above, understanding current processes is essential when considering implementation of a new automated system. How data is collected, stored, and accessed is important to understand. Use tools and gain a clear understanding of how things flow now, and what the expected flow will become.

3. Advanced analytics and decision automation – Vital when you consider both the business and clinical aspects of the medical practice. Inside the system, the detection and protection tools can be developed and made operational.

4. Cohesive, timely and flexible infrastructure – data storage, new and improved interfaces, and access to vendor(s), as well as the staff to ensure operational stability, are key.

5. Smart visualization – intuitive design, interactive, and personalized dashboard reporting is also key.

6. External ecosystem – working with external sources for patient portals, etc. will help prevent intrusion into your system.

7. Talent and culture – hiring and retaining the right staff with the technical, and personal communication skills, will ensure that the risks are being evaluated, prevented, reported, and hopefully stopped.

With all this said, a few steps that can be followed to ensure success in management of your current, and whatever new technology advances you choose to implement in your practice, are:

- Pick the right staff – refer to point seven above. Selection of the right skill level, and development of a trusting relationship in the IT area, is critical. As the first step, it is key to train staff throughout the practice, limiting and understanding proper use of internet access, scheduling training at onboarding, as well as at least annually, and so on. Following several of the steps noted relate to the learning organization within the context of the expanding digital world.
- Update equipment – review, on at least an annual basis, the equipment needs. As Moore's law notes, prices decrease, and new technology will change at least every two years. Keeping these improvements in mind during annual budget time is essential.
- Update per direction of software vendors – ensure that all updates are installed timely and completely. If additional training is required, schedule and follow through with that.
- Secure your network(s) – passwords, backup, firewalls, and following the detection, protection, and response protocols developed in your planning efforts will reduce the risk issues that surround your system.

The simpler you can make your comprehensive approach, the better. This may sound counter intuitive, but any system is only as strong as its weakest link. We do not intend to be a comprehensive instructional on technology, as things change too quickly. Hopefully we have, at least, challenged you to think through your needs of today, as well as for the foreseeable future.

The key point to remember from the chapter is we have only identified the tip of the ice berg. Accepting that technology offers benefits in clinical and business operations is key. Keeping up with these changes requires an investment in hardware, software, and processes to ensure adequate data, security, and efficiency. This cannot be done by one individual; it requires a team, and an investment in learning!

REFERENCES

1. https://en.wikipedia.org/wiki/Technology. Accessed December 1, 2018
2. Regalado A. We Need a Moore's Law for Medicine, *MIT Technology Review*. September 3, 2013. https://www.technologyreview.com/s/518871/we-need-a-moores-law-for-medicine/. Accessed December 1. 2018
3. Sahni, N et. al. The IT Transformation Health Care Needs, *Harvard Business Review*, Nov/Dec 2017. https://hbr.org/2017/11/the-it-transformation-health-care-needs
4. https://en.wikipedia.org/wiki/Blockchain. Accessed December 1, 2018
5. Kharpal A. Steven Hawking Says AI Could be the Worst Event in the History of our Civilization. Tech Transformers, a CNBC Special Report, November 6, 2017. https://www.cnbc.com/2017/11/06/stephen-hawking-ai-could-be-worst-event-in-civilization.html. Accessed December 1, 2018.
6. Skinner J. The Costly Paradox of Health Care Technology, *MIT Technology Review*, September 5, 2013. https://www.technologyreview.com/s/518876/the-costly-paradox-of-health-care-technology/. Accessed December 1, 2018.

7. Topol E. *The Creative Destruction of Medicine*, New York, NY: Basic Books; 2012.
8. McKinsey&Company: The Future of Risk Management in the Digital Era. https://www.mckinsey.com/business-functions/risk/our-insights/the-future-of-risk-management-in-the-digital-era. Accessed December 1, 2018.

RISK ASSESSMENT TOOL

Go to: https://www.ffiec.gov/pdf/cybersecurity/FFIEC_CAT_May_2017.pdf

Chapter 10

Your Practice Transition Roadmap

Up to this point, the book topics have focused on specific processes in the business of medical practice. From here, the focus will shift to how you can update, and improve, these processes to survive, and thrive.

The title "transition" was chosen to emphasize that there is more than a simple change required, as you consider applying the information shared here. Change in many dictionaries is defined as "make or become different."[1] This word is often overused, causes concerns, and brings resistance in the minds of leadership and staff. My 88-year old uncle recently shared an insight. He referenced the adage from Ben Franklin, that there are two things certain in life - death and taxes. My uncle believed it needed the addition of one more thing - change.

Given the connotation of change, let's focus on the word - transition. The definition from the same source is "the process or a period of changing from one state or condition to another."[2] I much prefer this term to change, since it talks about two key aspects of the management of the future – process, and period (of time) that requires changing to another.

Earlier, we contrasted the terms management and leadership. Revisiting them in terms of transition, we find

- Management is related to the tools or structures intended to control the "change"
- Leadership is the focus on the vision, processes, and driving forces that fuel the process of "change"[3]

In the beginning of the book, we focused on an honest assessment of your medical practice. Further in, we focused on the key aspects of planning. Based upon your analysis, what do you want to transition in your practice?

Before you answer, consider three levels of transition:

1. Straight forward – like when your Smart phone sends an update alert. The change is mostly behind the scenes and may not impact the entire phone. Perhaps you'd like to transition to add or delete an ancillary service? That action may or may not impact your entire core business.

2. Mindset – this is like when your Smart phone has added several features, which you think you will enjoy. You must read about them, understand them, and then decide

to implement them. Or, you may change software systems requiring significant efforts to train and implement.

3. Transformation – this example is when you move from Apple to Samsung. Or, you become integrated into another structure, and you add several specialists to your existing practice.[4]

Each of these levels of transition requires a different approach, and a different amount of effort, to achieve success.

Further conceptualization suggests that your change will be motivated by finances, or by the focus or ability of the organization itself to succeed. A financial perspective would require layoffs, a cancellation of a major payer contract, loss of a division, or something that requires significant effort. Even more direct, perhaps this involves a Theory X approach to achieving the outcome.

The organizational perspective focuses on the culture, structure, capabilities, skills, etc. that exist in the organization. A recent revised organizational structure, announced by Intermountain Health, is a good example. The shift moved from a regional organizational structure to one that separates primary care, and outpatient from specialists and inpatient. A theory Y approach may be appropriate here. There may not be significant technical changes, but the focus and culture of the organization will change and require both leadership commitment, and management expertise.

PHASES OF TRANSITION

William Bridges has championed that idea of transition in his book *Managing Transitions, Making the Most of Change*[5] He identifies a three-phase approach to managing transition. His phases are end, neutral zone, and beginning. The suggestion is to stop what has been TW^{2}ADI and move to a period of learning; accept the beginning of a new way of doing things. This is like Kurt Lewin's change theory, which also has three phases – unfreeze, freeze, and re-freeze.

The End phase is "letting go," and addresses several key points:
- Who's doing what – who is going to have to let go of something?
- Accept reality and importance of the losses
- Don't be surprised by the staff reaction
- Allow for acknowledgement of the loss
- Compensate for losses – don't just talk, but identify what is new compared to what is lost, and how things will improve

The neutral zone phase can be chaotic. Emotions will run higher with increased anxiety, absenteeism, and real resistance. This is the time to capitalize on this chaos by communication, educating, and seeking mutually beneficial outcomes. Create short wins, temporary solutions, and recognize/ reward even the smallest effort to transition to the new way.

The beginning is the actual implementation of the new way of doing things. This requires consistency, follow up, reinforcement, listening to those impacted to ensure that it works, tweaking the process based upon feedback, and monitoring the process to full implementation.

THE TRANSITION PROCESS

The key to success in any organization is the focus on its purpose - why do you exist, what is your vision, mission, and what are your values? Without these firmly in place and clearly understood by all, the practice will not succeed.

Reflect again on the first paragraph of this chapter, where you identified an area where a transition to a new way of doing things is necessary. What level of transition will you expect from your discovery? Basic, transformational or somewhere in between? Leadership must be behind this transition, and clearly understand the why and what to the move. Without leadership commitment, and a clear focus on the purpose and values, any effort will result in failure, frustration, and the inability to implement any future transitions.

There are a few key steps in the transition planning process that are necessary:
- What is the goal of the change?
  - Business case – financial, patient satisfaction, employee productivity improvement
  - Specifically define, key for future communication and measurement of success
- What is the time frame to make the transition?
  - How urgent is the matter?
- Who will be involved in developing the new way? (Team members!)
  - Process owners – involvement by those that do it now, and who will have the biggest impact of the transition
  - Management – someone to make sure the process flows smoothly
  - Facilitator – guidance from outside of the actual team, if necessary
- What communication models and frequency will be used, and what training process will be implemented?
  - Create a story about the change, to clearly illustrate the why, what, when, and the how all being asked, and answered, in the process
  - Expected benefits for the practice, the patient, and WIFM – what's in it for me (the staff member)
  - Written
  - Verbal
  - Listen
  - Demonstration
  - How many times will the story be repeated? Use the shampoo method - lather, rinse, repeat - until the message is clearly understood and accepted
- What resources will be required?

- What is the best approach to implementation and success?

In managing the transition process, two key aspects must be considered. First is the intellectual side. This is the explanation of the why, what, when, how, etc. and is the content of the policy/procedure change, and the content of the training program. The goal here is to appeal to the staff member's intellect, understanding, and rational being.

The second aspect is the emotional side. This is the most difficult aspect, and very often most overlooked. Daniel Goleman's 1995 book, *Emotional Intelligence* highlighted five domains of emotional intelligence, his acronym of EQ.[6] In short, the five domains are:

- Know your emotions
- Manage your own emotions
- Motivate yourself
- Recognize and understand other people's emotions
- Manage relationships, the emotions of others.

To put this all into context, refer to Figure 10-1 which identifies the ebb and flow of emotions over time when considering the phases of achieving a successful transition:

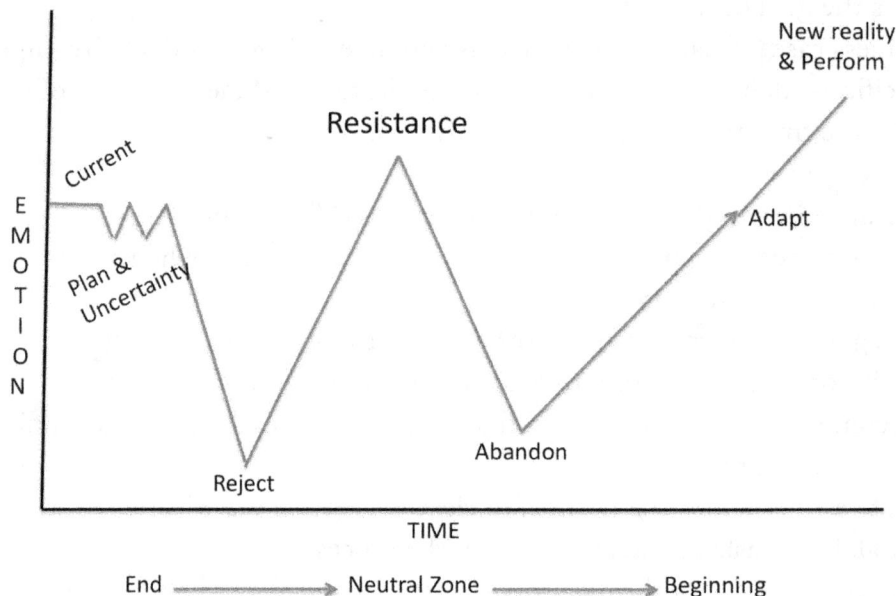

FIGURE 10-1. Emotion/Time

Assume that the current emotional state is level, and about mid-range on the scale. A need is identified which, when announced, creates a level of uncertainty. If the efforts at transition have not succeeded, the level of anxiety will increase, or resignation will set in, creating skepticism. It is at this point that the plan must be considered and fully developed.

Involving staff in the process is key here to help with awareness, identifying options for improvement, and setting the tone for successful implementation.

As you address the issues noted in the 'end' phase, and move to the neutral zone, the transition becomes more real, and the resistance emotion takes hold. It is possible to mediate the resistance emotion. However, there will be attempts to stop, or abandon, the change. If this occurs again, emotions will decrease, since it will not be a reality, or a reality they care about.

With involvement in development, repeated communication efforts and approaches, and adequate training through coaching and mentoring, the transition moves into the beginning phase and adaption sets in. Finally, performance, stability, and the new reality are accepted. A key, though, is to continue to follow through. As the chart depicts, hopefully the emotional aspect with improved outcomes results in higher emotional buy in by the staff, helping the new way exceed the targeted goals.

There are several emotions that could have been added to the figure, such as:

- Anxiety – this transition is out of my control, what will happen?
- Happiness – yes, the desired transition may result in happiness on the part of the staff.
- Fear – what will this mean? Will I lose my job? What if I can't do it the new way?
- Threat – I could lose my job, or someone else may be better at the new way. This could cause a major life style change for the individual.
- Guilt – have I not done things right, or why do they want to change my job? I must have really messed up.
- Depression – I don't want to do this, it will cause me problems. I'm depressed.
- Disillusionment – we've tried this before, or the practice goals are changing and are different than mine.
- Hostility – this won't work, and I'll make sure it doesn't.
- Denial – not accepting and denying that it will happen.

The most prevalent emotion is resistance. Table 10-1 from Kotter and Schlesinger in *Harvard Business Review*, identifies approaches to manage resistance.[7]

WHAT DOES THIS ALL MEAN?

With this information, you must assess your practice and its willingness to transition. Our discussion on scenario planning explored one scenario where the choice is to stay the same. This is surely a way to lead to retirement, sale, or closure of your practice. This may not always be bad. But it is important to note that if any of those options occur, you personally will undergo significant transition to a new way of life. There is no guarantee that this will be a positive move. Preparing for it will at least set a positive tone.

A simple way to gain an understanding about you personally is to move your desk, your work station, your pictures on the wall, or something that you touch or see regularly. How

TABLE 10-1. Managing Resistance to Transition

Approach	Commonly Used	Advantages	Disadvantages
Education + Communication	Where there is a lack of information or inaccurate information and analysis	Once persuaded, people will often help with the implementation of the change	Can be very time consuming if lots of people are involved
Participation+ Involvement	Where the initiators do not have all the information they need to design the change, and where others have considerable power to resist	People who participate will be committed to implementing change, and any relevant information they have will be integrated into the change plan	Can be very time consuming if participants design an inappropriate change
Facilitation+ Support	Where people are resisting because of adjustment problems	No other approach works as well with adjustment problems	Can be time consuming, expensive, and still fail
Negotiation + Agreement	Where someone or some group will clearly lose out in a change, and were that group has considerable power to resist	Sometimes it is a relatively easy way to avoid major resistance	Can be too expensive in many cases if it alerts other to negotiate for compliance
Manipulation + Co-optation	Where other tactics will not work or are too expensive	It can be a relatively quick and inexpensive solution to resistance problems	Can lead to future problems if people feel manipulated
Explicit + Implicit Coercion	Where speed is essential, and the change initiators possess considerable power	It is speedy and can overcome any kind of resistance	Can be risky if it leaves people mad at the initiators

does it feel when you experience this new thing? Seriously, think about doing this, and identifying your thoughts and feelings.

One thing we see frequently is the practice's board meeting deciding to change, and the next day a mandatory reaction to it. Take for example if 15 physician owners of the practice meet the third Tuesday of each month. The review of the financial, and other reports is routine. One member brings up a new treatment approach to patients who present with a certain disease state, and makes a recommendation concerning an evidence-based care plan. Discussion follows amongst the physician owners. A vote is taken, and it is unanimously decided to implement the new approach, with the effective start date the following Monday.

The staff is then informed, and necessary training and tools are developed. Then, you have a patient who presents as outlined, and the staff reminds you of the new way to approach. Your response is no, and that the others can do it that way, but you are not. This illustrates a passive aggressive response to a decision you were part of making. What message does this send to your staff? What have you done to undermine the group function? Awareness of the role of board member and practicing physician as two separate functions is key. Decision making like this is essential but follow up action is as well. Transitioning to a new way of doing things is not always easy but is necessary.

Employees, as well, who are set in their ways, TW²ADI. These can create issues of accountability and support. They can become informal leaders, undermining any transition effort. They can resist in many ways. Education and awareness of the benefits, holding them accountable for action, and in some cases, taking the most negative employee and placing them in charge of leading the transition, will work wonders in improving patient care. Improving patient care remains the goal.

Moving away from the negative implications, transition can be very positive. There are always new ways of doing things. Why do you need a front desk, when you have patient portals and tablets? Telemedicine and wearables offer ways to keep in touch with patients without a visit to the office. In population health and value-based payment modeling like capitation, these types of quick, insightful ways to reach the patient may be very effective.

Consider what kind of transitions have occurred in healthcare that you may, or may not, have been involved:

- Join ACO
- Sell practice to health system
- Join another practice
- Reduce staff, reduction in force
- EHR!
- Another software update
- New staff members, replacing old
- Revising job descriptions
- Consultant report and recommendations
- Payment changes
- Reduced revenue per contracts that you could not stop
- Increased patient payment responsibility
- Development and acceptance of clinical guidelines
- HIPAA and other rules
- PQRS, Meaningful Use, MIPS, APM
- Provider leaving
- New provider joining

- Founding physician leader retires
- Sudden death or injury of a provider
- Hurricane, flood
- Your own list

This should act as a teaser and is worth reviewing in terms of your practice. How did you do? What could have been done differently? Do not dwell on past changes as places of contention, but instead as teachable moments.

The development of a learning organization culture, and openness to innovation, require a transition to something different. This different approach is what has an impact on decision making, investments, and choosing the right scenario. The attitude that innovation, transformation, increased efficiency to ensure more access, contributes to the growth of the business makes sense. These cannot be done by TW^{2}ADI!

REFERENCES

1. https://en.oxforddictionaries.com/definition/change. Accessed December 1, 2018
2. https://en.oxforddictionaries.com/definition/transition. Accessed December 1, 2018
3. Kotter J. Change Management vs. Change Leadership – What's the Difference? *Forbes*, July 12, 2011. https://www.forbes.com/sites/johnkotter/2011/07/12/change-management-vs-change-leadership-whats-the-difference/#514427c24cc6. Accessed December 1, 2018.
4. Lawson E, Price C. The Psychology of Change Management, *McKinsey Quarterly*, June 2003. https://www.mckinsey.com/business-functions/organization/our-insights/the-psychology-of-change-management. Accessed December 1, 2018.
5. Bridges W. *Managing Transitions, Making the Most of Change*, Boston, MA: DaCapo Lifelong Books; 2003.
6. Goleman D. *Emotional Intelligence*, New York, NY: Bantam Books; 1995
7. Kotter P, Schlesinger L. Choosing Strategies for Change, *Harvard Business Review*, July-August 2008. https://hbr.org/2008/07/choosing-strategies-for-change. Accessed December 1, 2018

CHANGE MANAGEMENT SURVEY

	Yes	No
1. I think the changes that are happening are for the best		
2. I need to make the best of change		
3. I obstruct the changes that are taking place		
4. I feel angry about the changes		
5. I'd prefer to stay as we were before the change		
6. I am prepared to help other accept change		
7. There might be benefits to be gained from change		
8. I withhold my support for change		
9. I am anxious about change		
10. I don't want to know about change		
11. My workplace will be better as a result of change		
12. I am willing to find out more about change and how it will affect me		
13. I blame management		
14. I feel frustrated that I have no control over change		
15. If I ignore change, it might not affect me		
16. I feel committed to change		
17. Change is not as bad as I originally thought		
18. I openly resist change		
19. I am upset at the need to change		
20. I can't believe that change is for the good		
21. I can see the benefits of change		
22. I accept the need to change		
23. I make my complaints known about change		
24. I feel sad at the loss of status quo		
25. I'd rather get on with what I am doing then to be involved in change		
26. We will benefit positively from change that is happening		
27. I have started to explore what change means to me		
28. I am looking for other work possibilities that are not affected by change		
29. I feel emotional about losing our old ways of working		
30. Change won't affect me		

Scoring

Put a checkmark by each statement number where you scored "yes." Then total the number of checkmarks in each column.

1._____   2. _____   3. _____   4. _____   5._____

6._____   7. _____   8. _____   9. _____   10._____

11._____   12. _____   13. _____   14. _____   15._____

16._____   17. _____   18. _____   19. _____   20._____

21._____   22. _____   23. _____   24. _____   25._____

26._____   27. _____   28. _____   29. _____   30._____

C_____   A _____   R _____   E _____   D_____

Source: *Compendium of Questionnaires and Inventories, Vol. 1*, Sarah Cook

Chapter 11

The Opportunity for Practice Transformation

I t is vital to acknowledge that transition is a way of life; there is a need to change the way we do things. A good example of this in the medial field is the development of the retail clinic model. This model was created by someone outside of healthcare who identified a need and developed a solution. Another example is the evolution of technology into the medical field in the form of wearables, insideables, and telemedicine. These are examples of innovative ways to accomplish the goals in the physician office, with fresh approaches.

Why is Amazon, Berkshire Hathaway, and many others exploring avenues into healthcare delivery? Is it because we, in the medical world, have failed? Or, is it because they think they can do it better? Consider the CVS – Aetna merger, which brings something new to the table. They can better control costs, better use technology, and be more efficient in order to deliver a more cost-effective service — at least that's their claim. But, do they have a point? The point is that if we, in the industry, do not respond more effectively, we may be the next employee of Amazon.

As mentioned with the development of the retail clinic model, there are changes occurring in the overall delivery model. We now have ACOs, to evolving free standing emergency rooms, to urgent care centers, to options for long term care. While these are important to be aware of, it is important to continually monitor what is going on in your local market. The practice question is, "what can you do inside of your practice's four walls?"

Here is a great quote from Accenture consulting:[1]

"Expanding markets, increasing global competition, rising customer expectations, advanced technologies, increasing digitization—every change in the market affects how a company operates and performs, often dramatically. And these days, it is difficult to respond to one disruption before being thrown off course by the next one.

Exceptionally savvy companies manage these changes by developing broad, cohesive, end-to-end global operating strategies that enable profitable growth and staying nimble enough to respond to rapidly-changing conditions—strategies that not just account for the power of technology to drive innovation but thrive on it."

The global healthcare system is fragmented, or siloed, usually with one specialist not always knowing what another specialist is doing. And the same can be said for the inner workings of the practice. The front desk doesn't know, or sometimes doesn't care, what is happening in the clinic, and vice versa. These silos must be removed both externally (integrated medical record) and internally (engaging, cross training, and talking to each other.)

Let's identify what transformation means, and what it involves. A recent article in the *Harvard Business Review* identified three different categories of effort.[2]

- Operational – doing things cheaper, faster, and better than what has been done previously. There could be improvements in efficiency, like seeing one more patient per day, or in-patient satisfaction, but this does not represent a major change in the business model. These improvements are not wrong, but instead could be a great place to start to help develop, and evolve, a culture of change and transformation. Think Lean and Six Sigma.

- Operational Model – seeing patients, but in a totally different way. Think about Netflix, and when the company shifted from mailing DVDs to online delivery of the same plus providing improved and original content. Also consider what happened to Blockbuster. An example in the medical world are the retail clinics and urgent care centers vs. the good old 15 minute per visit schedule. Think Lean and Six Sigma.

- Strategic – The example we can use here is of Walgreens. This company went from a drug store, to retail, to managing chronic diseases. In the medical world, the practice that has a 50% patient population with Hepatitis C, or the oncology practice that sees the evolution of oral chemotherapy drugs, could plan strategic growth around what they identify as the need. Think reengineering.

The need for personal care and no wait time will always be present, but what about introducing new technology to meet these needs like robots, wearables, and the walk-in complete body scan? Or, financially, what if you considered a shift from fee-for-service to value-based, bulk payments. And still yet, a shift from sick care to well care. What will you need to do to survive, and thrive, with all these new ideas evolving?

Can you think of ways to change by not TW²ADI, and come up with a new and better way? Always keep in mind what could be a NWTDI - New Way To Do It! Why do we need a reception desk, when we can use kiosks? Or instead, how about using tablets to greet patients, complete with pictures, demographic and insurance information, reason for visit, and a credit card reader? After the initial check in with the tablet, the patient could be greeted and escorted to an exam room set up for triage. This would eliminate the need for waiting rooms, and instead, all that space could be converted to additional exam rooms. Or, when the patient arrives in the parking lot, they slide their ID card, check in, pay, and are told to go to an exam room, where they are cheerfully greeted by a staff member. Even more advanced, what if, as they walk into the office, a scanner built into the door frame runs all vitals? Who knows what is possible; let your imagination run away with your thoughts in order to find new options for innovation.

Why are you in business? To take care of the patient! What does the patient, or customer, want, or need? Do they want reliability, speed, attentiveness to their concerns, solutions to their state of health, confirmation that they are doing well, or effective management of their chronic condition? Any, or all, of these are critical. The point is that, when you think of transformation, start with what the customer wants, or needs, and rethink where you are in meeting those needs.

Not everything needs to be solved with implementing new technological resources. Earlier we referred to a work done by Clayton Christensen, *The Innovator's Prescription*. He noted that there are several types of patient visits, including the need for diagnosis (acute), to treatment (surgery, infusion), to chronic to wellness. In most offices, these four types of patients are seen throughout any one day. Stopping and analyzing the data may reveal that there are bottlenecks, caused by one type over another. Perhaps there is a better way, better time, or better provider (special interest of one provider, mid-level support) to see patients of this type. This could result in some interesting transformative approaches to dealing with those bottlenecks in a more efficient, and effective way.

In the finance chapter, we talked about budgeting. How about starting the next budget period with the idea of zero-based budgeting? This was a big focus a few years ago in many industries and is becoming popular once again. This idea challenges you to start with a clean slate - no employees, no supplies, and no equipment. Instead, you simply explore what you need in an area (front desk, triage) to provide the service to the patient in the most efficient way possible? Build the budget based upon the outcome of that discussion, rather than based upon what the revenue and expenses were last year. This may offer an open transformative look at the practice model.

Transformation needs to start somewhere. It does not necessarily need to result in a major change immediately, but instead, minor steps to meet the needs of the customers can be powerful. Let's refer to the ISO discussion. ISO 9001:2015 sets a great tone for quality improvements in Clause 8, Operations. The framework is outlined in Figure 11-1. We have adapted it to a framework for innovation.

At the top we see 8.3.2, or Planning. This refers to identifying a need for improvement. This can be done by Gemba, walking to the area, response from patient satisfaction surveys, identified wastes, errors, hassle factors, or employee input. This step involves detecting something that needs improvement and identifying an opportunity.

In 8.3.3, we look at the Inputs. What are the activities, or steps taken, to accomplish the task, or move through the tasks in the process? Here, data, or brainstorming, can open new ideas. You can break the mold, re-engineer, or think out of the box. This, again, cannot be

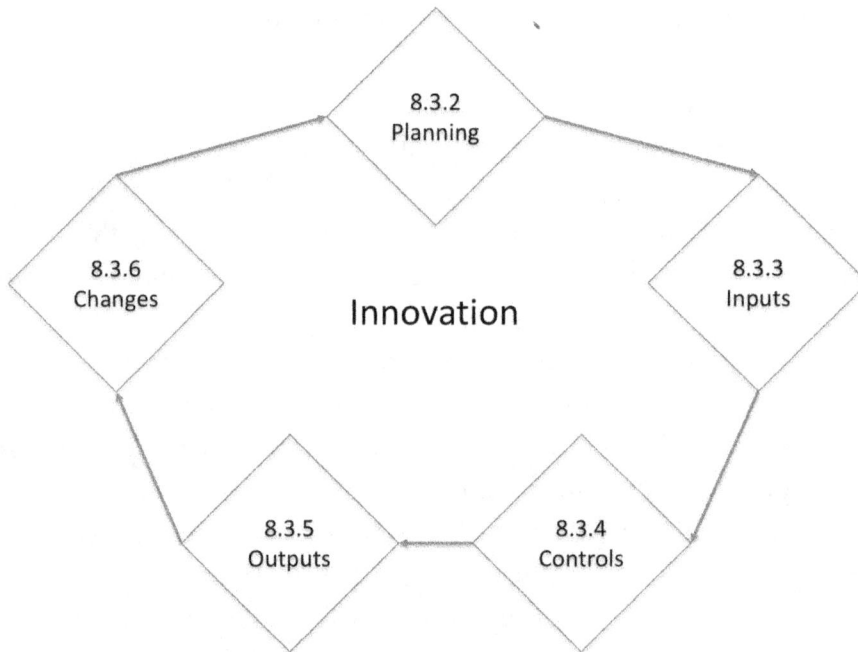

FIGURE 11-1. ISO 9001:2015 Operations

done by one individual. In this step, process owners (those that do the work), and those who have inputs, can have unrestricted review, and opportunity to create ideas.

8.3.4 speaks to Control, which is where the ideas developed through inputs are reduced to one. You design a pilot test and select an area to experiment with the new way of doing things. Don't' be afraid of this step and consider the statements all over the internet that suggest "fail early, fail fast, fail often"! The point is that, if you don't try something, nothing new will result. If the pilot test fails, it will be early enough to try again. Continual failure may make little sense, but the important part is that it has been tried.

Once the pilot test has been revised to achieve a new, and better way of doing things, you have come to 8.3.5, or the Outputs. Here, you have arrived to where you can go back to the source, or the customer, and determine if it really works, and meets the original hypothesis. Here, you must keep it simple and verify your results.

8.3.6 is labeled by ISO as Change. Hopefully, we have now arrived at a transformed process that improves the results experienced by the customer. Memorialize the NWTDI in your formal policies and procedures, training manual and program, and implement it practice wide.

Another question about transformation is whether you have the organizational structure, the KSA (knowledge, skills, and attitude) team, to make it happen. Can your organization move quickly and easily? Are you agile enough to respond, and lead into the future?

What is the source of the idea, or the concept, desired? Is the plan original and new, e.g., mid-level supported clinics in retail settings for the convenience of the patient? Or, is the idea something being done by other local practices, or in other markets? Many studies do reveal that improving on an idea, rather than being the first mover, has long term benefits.

One approach to transforming the practice is to plan, plan, plan, and then execute. Much of the time should be spent in reviewing and considering, and then implementing. This proves to be a valid approach in some cases, with some teams, and in some organizations. The steps are simple:

- Define, or identify, the opportunity
- Review resources required to make it happen, and what is needed to secure, shift, train, or other action. A repeated key here is to involve others, as transformation does not come from you. Instead, it requires other ideas, and buy in, to achieve success.
- Develop the implementation approach
- Implement

Another approach is to follow what has been done in developing software programs using iterative development. The application here is for when the project is large, and why this approach is often used in software development. Basically, it breaks down in these steps:

- Design
- Develop
- Test
- Repeat (until the total goal is reached)

A recent McKinsey article pointed out key areas to watch out for when doing a transformation:

1. Ensure alignment with key stakeholders and ensure the value of the transformation.
   a. Very often a new way to do it, NWTDI, is the idea of one person and the sale of the idea, development of approach, etc. is not well thought out.
   b. Get everyone involved to see the true benefit and encourage input to identify the true value to your customer.
2. Go beyond simple pilot tests in setting priorities.
   a. It is always good when developing a new, or improved, concept to test it out.
   b. Recognize what the pilot test is, and that moving the new concept throughout the organization requires significant thought and effort.
3. Culture must come first.
   a. It has been said that culture eats strategy; apply that to a new idea.
   b. If the culture is not there to accept and support something, other than TW^{2}ADI, it is doomed to fail.
4. Utilize the talents of others.

    a. Level 5 leadership suggests that working with others, and not taking full responsibility or credit for a transformation, is a winner.

    b. Involve those that do the work will be impacted the most by the new concept.

    c. They may have more ideas or will see the pitfalls of the discussion. When it's time to implement, they will be committed to make it happen.

5. Identify the scale, and scope, of the impact of the transformation.

    a. Many will wonder why the project hasn't been completed already.

    b. Working on a transformation is very different than seeing a patient, where determining what is wrong, and implementing a course of treatment, can all happen in only 15 minutes.

    c. The scale and scope will help determine the process of implementation, revision, and follow up, as well as set expectations.

6. Have solid infrastructure and commitment.

    a. Practices fail due to poor infrastructure.

    b. Practices fail when all are not committed to its overall mission.

    c. This remains the same for any transformation.

7. Does the DNA support transformation?

    It is critical to accept the fact that change is inevitable, whether leading or following, and the organization must be committed to it.

Another McKinsey article noted survey results of what are keys to success in transformation. Table 11-1.[3] These relate to the idea that employee engagement, and associated activities, are critical to the successful transformation in any organization.

Consider this great example of how to go about transforming your practice: very often we see a problem with no-shows. The first reaction is to penalize the patient with a fee if they do not show. This not only creates a public relations issue but also creates an issue in managing the revenue cycle. The second response is to robot call, text, or email two or three times to remind the patient of their appointment time.

Instead, it is important to take a serious look at some of the things that may create this problem:

- Scheduling model – set up for the physician rather than the patient, e.g., no early morning or late afternoon options for working patients.
- Acute vs. chronic patient needs.
- Payer analysis – more patients that require authorizations, or have certain insurances, are more likely to be no shows. Perhaps working with the payer and their support system may help.
- Doctors always running behind by greater than 30 minutes.
- Distance between call for appointment, or the actual appointment.
- Which day of the week, or time of day, has more no shows?

TABLE 11-1. Keys to Successful Transformation

Actions Taken	Approaches to Employee Engagement
Leaders ensure that frontline staff felt ownership for the change	The transformation was organized into a clear structure with readily understandable sections
Roles and responsibilities were clear, so people felt accountable through ongoing communications and involvement	Clear, unambiguous metrics and milestones were in place to ensure that progress and impact were rigorously tracked
Our best talent was deployed to carry out the most critical parts of the transformation	The right information was available at the right time for managers to monitor the transformation's progress and troubleshoot where required.
Leader role-modeled the desired change	

Exploring these factors allow us to consider alternative transformation options to help fix the problem. If you have many chronic disease patients, will group visits work? How about more follow up calls, and utilization of the chronic care codes? How about use of transition care codes for those who are discharged. Looking at patient engagement, and showing concern for their care, may be enough to eliminate no shows. Of course, the other option is for chronic no shows, terminate them from the practice with the 30-day letter (approved by your malpractice carrier).

The point in this example is to highlight the need to really understand the reasons for an issue, rather than throwing something out that is a simple, quick solution. There are solutions. Engaging the patient, calling to monitor their treatment plan progress, using technology, open access scheduling (same day), and the like may all be realistic alternative solutions. These don't seem transformative, but the transformation part is taking a serious look at the etiology to understand, rather than just offer a quick fix.

But this is not the end. Any transformation program requires follow up. This means setting a time frame, e.g., monthly or three months, to review this transformed way of doing things, in order to ensure that the results are solid. If they are not, there is no problem in revising the areas that are not working to meet your expectations. Don't stop working towards transformation; always keep moving forward.

REFERENCES

1. Operations and Process Transformation, Accenture. https://www.accenture.com/us-en/service-operations-process-transformation-overview. Accessed December 1, 2018.

2. Anthony S. What Do You Really Mean By Business "Transformation"? *Harvard Business Review*, February 26, 2016; https://hbr.org/2016/02/what-do-you-really-mean-by-business-transformation. Accessed December 1. 2018.

3. What Successful Transformations Share: McKinsey Global Survey Results. McKinsey. https://www.mckinsey.com/business-functions/organization/our-insights/what-successful-transformations-share-mckinsey-global-survey-results. Accessed December 1, 2018.

SYSTEMS THINKING TRANSFORMATION TOOL

- The core that got you here
  - Purpose – heroism, altruism, discovery, excellence
  - Identity – brand
  - Long range intention
- The context that got you here
  - Create goals
  - Measurements
  - Systems
  - Organizational structure
  - Technology
  - Strategy
- The capability that got you here
  - Translate – goals, metrics, structure, and strategy
  - Need prioritization and resource allocation
- The competency that got you here
  - 10,000 hours of relevant experience
- The capacity that got you here
  - Right amounts
- The customer outcome that got you here
  - Transform = serve in a new way
- The culture that got you here
  - How things get done – way goals set, measurements selected
  - Observing how people do what they do
  - Change culture by changing all of the above

What got you here may kill you

1. Do you know what made you successful? How do you know?
2. What strengths do you have that are now liabilities?
3. What is the difference between our brand today and what you must make your brand stand out in the future?
4. How must the core of the enterprise change?
5. How must the context of the enterprise change?
6. What fundamental capabilities must the organization acquire?
7. In what way must the culture change moving forward?
8. Have you remapped the metrics to encourage the right action?
9. Have you removed the pathology of "do it all"?
10. Have you made the entire investment in transformation or only part of it?

Yesterday's leadership skills

1. What is your point of view on leadership? Does it match the reality of the challenges you face?
2. What leadership strengths from the past are now weaknesses?
3. What new leadership competencies are critical to your transformation?
4. Where are your potential blind spots in terms of leadership competencies?
5. What changes are you willing to make in leadership to be successful in transformation?
6. Do you have superior listening strength?
7. What is your tolerance for ambiguity?
8. Have you specifically looked at the level of narcissism in the organization?
9. Do you and your team have solid self-awareness? How do you know?
10. Is the transformation of the organization really your thing?

There is no strategy if nobody knows what to do

1. Can your organization state your strategy consistently in plain language?
2. Is you ask five people at random what the company strategy is, will they answer consistently, coherently, and correctly?
3. What is the success rate of your projects? How do you know?
4. Is your strategy more than a statement of financial measurements?
5. Has the team been immersed in strategy, or was it handed to them?
6. Are you willing to invest in ensuring that strategy is deeply understood in the organization?
7. Has the strategy been translated into an investment portfolio of projects to make it happen?
8. Are the resources available to accomplish the strategy? How do you know?
9. Can you draw a picture of your goals and strategy freehand on a single piece of paper? Can your team do the same?
10. Do you have a way of tracing strategy to goals to measurements to projects to tasks and back again?
11. If you had to take a reduction of 20 percent, would you know what to cut so that you minimize the impact on your goals?

Transforming strategy

1. Has your organization installed tool or systems in the absence of a process that utilizes the tools effectively? (Have you become a fool with a tool?)
2. Does your organization suffer from system overkill for the problem at hand?
3. Do you have lots of data but no real information?
4. Does the executive team understand portfolio management?
5. Have you linked projects to goals?

6. Do you have a balanced and comprehensive decision-making system that goes beyond the obvious ROI criteria?
7. Do you have a strategic execution office that centralizes control over low-maturity processes?
8. What is the state of your project management capability?
9. Do you have internal champions who have the influence to create real change?
10. Are you willing to take the (your practice name) oath?
    a. As a member, I promise
        i. I will strive to act with honesty and integrity
        ii. I will respect the rights and dignity of all people
        iii. I will strive to create sustainable prosperity worldwide
        iv. I will oppose all forms of corruption and exploitation, and
        v. I will take responsibility for my actions
        vi. As I hold true to these principles, it is my hope that I may enjoy an honorable reputation and peace of conscience
        vii. This pledge I make freely and upon my honor

What are the factors that account for our success?
- Supply chain efficiency, design, dominance, exclusivity, and so on
- Distribution network size, design, alliances
- Vertical integration
- Defensible market position through differentiation
- Brand power
- The overall solution offered
- The creation of a system or platform
- Intellectual or emotional appeal
- Product or service features, function quality or performance
- Service

How do we know?
What do we have which shows that to be the case?

What are the future drivers of success that represent transformation
- Control of scarce resources
- Defensible technological position
- Solving more of the customer's problems
- Channel partners
- Consultative solutions

How do we know?
What do we have which shows that to be the case?

Transform Human resources

1. Is your HR organization a strategic advantage?
2. Have you got the right people on the bus for transformation?
3. Have your strategy and transformation been translated into HR requirements?
4. Is your HR organization getting the basic job done? Does it have the capability to lead transformation?
5. Does your HR organization have the capacity to take on a more strategic role?
6. If you are in an academic role, have you begun to change the way HR professionals are educated?
7. Are you are part of a professional association, have you begun to shift the conversation to be inclusive of organizational strategic planning, not just HR, and other related disciplines?
8. Has the organization taken on the challenge of putting A players in all key roles, starting at the top?
9. Do you develop HR professionals with rotational assignments so that they learn the business model?
10. How often has your HR organization been the driving force behind change?

	Goals	Transition	Management
Organization	What we will achieve together	Design of our path, team, and culture	Leader accountability
Process	What our processes must achieve	Processes to set priority and execute	Process accountability
Individual	What we must achieve individually	Skills, tools, and systems	Individual accountability

Chapter 12

The Culture of your Healthcare Practice: Putting the Pieces Together

There is a reason why is the discussion on culture has been kept until the end of the book. All the previous information leads to a serious review about what your culture is, and if you have the ability, willpower, and group identity to transition in the new world of healthcare. Furthermore, do you have the mission to continually seek to improve care, provided to your patients, over the long term?

Gary Kaplan, M.D. Chairman and CEO of Virginia Mason, in a webinar in the fall of 2017, offered a great quote that helps set the tone for the message of this chapter: "We had to challenge our old paradigms. Physicians are instrumental in setting the tone, and unless the physicians believe we're on the right path we don't have the kind of alignment that will help us move forward."[1] The tone set by leadership, and as noted by Kaplan by physicians, is critical, not only in setting the tone for culture, but all aspects necessary to be successful in the business world.

Let's start with a definition of the term culture, as defined in Edgar H. Schein's book, *Organization Culture and Leadership*. His formal definition is "defined as a pattern of shared basic assumptions learned by a group as it solved its problems of external adaptation and internal integration, which has worked well enough to be considered valid and, therefore, to be taught to new members as the correct way to perceive, think, and feel in relation to those problems."[2]

Schein, considered by many the authority on culture, suggests a key is the group, since there is some order, and a semblance of common direction, differing from the definition of a crowd. This is critical because a group, that has no common mission or direction, is more like a crowd, and is destined to break up in a short period of time.

The external adaptation noted in the definition relates to survival, and/or growth, as the group adapts to its environment. The internal integration relates to how the organization functions. The latter is key, and without a solid infrastructure it is impossible to survive in any external environment, as noted throughout this book.

Schein notes that culture is formed over time based upon the direction, or sense, from the founder(s) of the organization. Their initial plan, and direction, is based upon the vision and discussion, which leads to actions consistent with that vision. There are three key aspects of the culture development, and subsequent maintenance:

- Artifacts – external actions, signs, symbols, observed behavior, and words used by members of the group. External in the fact that they can be observed and do assist in framing.

- Espoused beliefs and values – group learning comes from someone's beliefs and values, typically starting with the founders. These become shared when the group accepts them through actions.

- Basic assumptions – these are solid, difficult to change, and built on the espoused values and beliefs established through group activities and norms of behavior. Focus, attention to details, meaning of actions and words, and emotions in situations form these assumptions. The mental models noted in the learning organization discussion are formed, and defined, by these basic assumptions.

Putting all these aspects together will create a perspective on how the culture works in your organization. In many groups, leadership will talk about one thing, while the artifacts tell a very different story. All groups state that their mission is to provide quality of care and meet the needs of patients. Yet, actions indicate that the real goal is to enhance the bottom line. This is demonstrated through examples like the compensation formula, decisions made on the treatment plan, human resource management (hire cheap, and fire whenever), and agreement at board meetings to change a policy without follow up action from all the doctors.

There are also groups that take this seriously and honor the quality of care initiative. These groups typically show actions like Board meeting discussions about effectiveness in compliance with treatment plans, a review of any safety issues last month, and the like. What should be noted here is that leadership from physician owners sets the tone by beliefs and values, which lead to assumptions noted by staff through the artifacts that are observed and experienced.

A recent article in the *Harvard Business Review* by Groysberg, et. al. identified eight different culture styles.[3] This is a result of a significant review of the literature and the experience of the authors. As you review this list, attempt to identify which one, or which ones, relate to your current organizational culture. There is no right or wrong answer. Instead, simply take an honest look at which style might define your practice.

- Caring – warm, sincere, relational
- Purpose – idealistic, tolerant, purpose driven
- Learning – open, inventive, exploring
- Enjoyment – playful, instinctive, fun loving
- Results – achievement, driven, goal focused
- Authority – bold, decisive, dominant

- Safety – realistic, careful, prepared
- Order – rule abiding, respectful, cooperative

Then, further intersperse each style with a framework that address stability vs. flexibility, and interdependence vs. independent. Stability reflects authority and safety, while flexibility reflects learning and purpose. Independence fits with enjoyment and results, while interdependence with caring and order.

As your read through these, you might think you are all of them, or you might think you're none of them, or maybe the framework does not fit your model. Their research shows that results and caring are the first two in the ranking. They appear to be opposite, since someone that is driven is not typically also caring. Instead, caring would seem to be perfect for a compassionate medical practice. But to explore this, just ask the simple question of what's more important at the monthly Board meeting: the financial statement, or quality/patient satisfaction. It is vital you are honest here.

Given the changing healthcare world with value-based payments and population health in the forefront, which of these styles best fits your practice? Is your purpose, as expressed in your mission statement, reflecting your practice today? Do you have fun at work, or are you facing burnout and too much stress? Is there one dominant personality that controls all decisions? In value-based care, are you safe, or a risk taker? Is everyone compliant?

Reflect on the discussion on your organization chart and your decision-making processes. Now consider the eight styles listed above. Where do you fit?

In our experience, we have seen mission statements that say one thing, yet the practice follows another road. If you look at your practice for culture, a valuable first look is at the compensation formula. A strict production formula, whether RVU, payment or other base, creates a result-oriented practice. More to the point, if you have 12 physicians, you may have 12 practices. Some may prefer safety (stability), while other prefer learning (flexibility), and still others prefer authority (stability).

One thing that should be obvious is if you don't control your culture, it will control you. Therefore, the key is to understand the culture and then, as suggested throughout this book, be prepared to change it as necessary to meet the ever-changing external environment. Put simply, if everyone in your practice continues to do things, or act, the way they do today, can you expect to survive, or grow, in the future? If the answer is yes, skip the rest of this chapter. If no, read on.

Step one is an honest assessment of your culture. What are the drivers of your culture addressing such things as compensation, decision making authority and timing, communication between and through all levels, staff accountability to policies and procedures, physician compliance with agreed upon care plans, risk tolerance, goals, reporting of data regularly, specifically, actionable vs simply informational which does not lead to compliance or appropriate actions, expenditures on facilities, training, uniforms, investment and use in and of technology, and so much more.

Once this is reviewed, the gaps and road blocks to achieving desired results will be obvious. The effort, then, should be directed toward fixing those issues and creating a new, or revised, culture. Achieving this new culture will not happen overnight and will require significant resources and time.

Practice leadership must take hold of the effort to revise or refine the culture. After the assessment, acceptance of where the issues are, and where the process should take hold, follows. As you reflect on the topics of this book, leadership must consider each one related to which style, or styles, represent the best fit. Culture change will take time, therefore, simply looking at the style list and checking off what applies, and what doesn't, will not work. It is important to have a serious discussion, one that results in 100% leadership buy in.

How are you going to make the revision happen? What type, and how often will there be communication? Refer to the learning chapter for additional thoughts on this. It's not enough to teach and communicate. The leadership must demonstrate commitment, without passive aggressive behavior.

The key is to hold yourselves, and all members of your team, accountable for actions that occur. Remember is it the experiences, either observed or impacted, that lead to the change in culture. You will want to work through a model that holds each individual accountable for their actions, as the new or revised culture evolves. The keys to accountability is to see, own, solve, and do the things necessary to comply with the culture change. This will lead to the desired results.

When you, or a team member, sees something that is counter to the desired norm, do you enable them to change? Does TW^{2}ADI rule the organization when they see something? The excuse that it has always been done that way will no longer work in the new culture. Holding staff accountable, but using these moments as either teachable, or as an encouragement for listening to new ideas, will prove as powerful toward effective culture change.

The team member who sees the action should then own it and accept responsibility to seek ways to improve. A culture must recognize the ability of a team member to identify, but also suggest or develop new ways to do things. Or, in the event of a culture change to identify an issue and come up with a better way to do things, to meet the goals of the new culture is a winner. This then solves the problem in concept.

This new idea communicated to leadership, and others on the team, must be to do, or adapt, to the new way of doing things.

As you explore this, consider what the new goals, as well as the desired results, may be:
- Move from fee-for-service to value-based payment, 50% year one, and expect 90% in three years
- Improve patient satisfaction scores to 95% "5s"
- Reduce turnover by 50%

These three goals may seem huge, and distinct, from each other, but if your practice sees the benefit of improved patient and staff engagement leading to reduced turnover and improved satisfaction the value-based payment move will benefit.

A transition plan is developed based upon the goals. This is done by a champion at the leadership level, teams (from key departments, as well as cross functional), communication on what the plan is, as well as throughout the process with key milestones expected and achieved, and patience. Any culture change will not occur instantly. Remember that it will take time. The staff is enabled, encouraged, informed, and able to openly share what they see through in making the positive changes and successful culture change.

One last thing to explore may be considered the elephant in the room. Are you are considering, or have recently, merged with a hospital, health system, or another medical group? What analysis was done related to culture? Where will you fit in? How are decisions made? What control will you have? Do you want control? If you are considering a merger, the above discussion is essential for serious review. If merged, take another look at what happens.

We have seen too many physicians give up, and choose to merge, without thinking through the above discussion. This has resulted in unhappiness, burnout, early retirement, or complacency in action. Obviously, this is not the desired outcome.

REFERENCES

1. MacDonald I. These 6 Healthcare Leaders Say Quality Improvement is an Organizational-Wide Effort and a Cultural Imperative. January 3, 2018. *FierceHealthcare.com*. https://www.fiercehealthcare.com/healthcare/6-inspiring-quotes-improving-quality-from-6-healthcare-leaders. Accessed December 1, 2018.
2. Schein E. *Organizational Culture and Leadership*, 4th Ed. San Francisco, CA: Josey-Bass; 2010
3. Groysberg B. et al. The Leader's Guide to Corporate Culture, *Harvard Business Review*, Jan/Feb 2018. https://hbr.org/2018/01/the-culture-factor

Chapter 13

Continuous Process Improvement (CPI) and Conclusion

Let's get technical. Although the title of this chapter is "continuous," we could have chosen "continual." W. Edwards Deming preferred using the term continual which he recognized as having many different approaches in different areas, to achieve improvement. Continuous has been referred to as a subset of continual. For our purposes here, we prefer continuous due to the implication that in your practice, t is an ongoing and constant effort, to improve processes.

Process as defined by dictionary.com is simply "a systematic series of actions directed to some end".[1] That's what happens all the time in your office, continuous activity to provide care, to submit an insurance claim, to hire a new employee, and so on. It is these processes that have been addressed in one way or another throughout this book.

The Japanese term for this concept is Kaizen, which is change for the better, in all aspects of life and the organization. Perhaps we have touched on points in this work that will have an impact on you both personally and professionally. Adapting a culture of improvement, regardless of your situation, will lead to the ultimate reason we choose to work in healthcare – to achieve satisfactory outcomes for every patient we encounter. Doing this through an efficient organization, treating staff members with respect and understanding, having the right staff members in place, and encouraging all to become part of the process will achieve the best targeted outcome possible.

Simply put, DO NOT REST ON TW²ADI! Always seek to improve. This requires a culture change in your practice. It requires leadership and management, it requires recognition that the practice exists to meet the needs of its customer (patient), utilizes resources all working together, applying business principles to be as efficient and effective as possible.

Hopefully you've been exposed to some new ideas and have been challenged to improve patient care by reading this book. Now you are prepared to think about developing your own master check list, or a series of check lists to help guide you on your own Continuous Process Improvement, CPI, strategy.

Atul Gawande, CEO of ABC (Amazon, Berkshire, and Chase) consortium, as well as physician, author/speaker, has championed the use of checklists in healthcare. His book, *The Checklist Manifesto: How to Get Things Right*, identified positive outcomes from the use of checklists.[2] The concept is mainly taken from the airline industry. Here are some checklists for you to consider in your own practice:

For the patient:
- Communication
- Evidence-based care plan
- Team approach; get everyone involved
- Engage patient in their own care
- Achieve comprehensive satisfaction scores

For the staff members:
- Select and retain the employees with the correct fit
- Engage all in the processes leading to successful
- Ensure effectiveness
- Evaluate and reward appropriately
- Start with YOU to accept the need to improve

For the supply chain and partners:
- Select the right partners
- Evaluate, at least annually, the cost/benefit of the relationship
- Seek others to expand or replace as necessary

For the business:
- Do an annual review
- Develop an annual business plan
- Update the plan
- Ensure the proper focus for care for the patient

For the efficient and effective process:
- Accept that improvements are necessary for the business
- Utilize the Lean and Six Sigma tools
- Develop an approach that achieves consistency in all processes from patient care to all aspects of support for the care provided

For the learning organization:
- Adopt a learning philosophy
- Include training and education in the budget
- Onboard
- Seek to improve EACH team member

For the finances:
- Accept the new model of bringing value through effective financial management, recording, and reporting
- Understand the entire operation, beyond the revenue cycle and look at the cost of providing services, each step along the way
- Annually review and update the benchmark data of the organization internally

For the technology:
- Accept the new
- Integrate new technologies into the business flow
- Protect the business from any cyber intrusion
- Develop the "people" talent necessary to optimize the investment in new technology

For transition:
- You are the first one to "change;" it starts with you
- Recognize the organization cannot be stagnant and that "change" is inevitable
- Develop a framework within which transition can consistently occur

For transformation:
- Don't be afraid to try something new
- The new model for delivering care includes all the above from learning to technology

For culture:
- Again, transition starts with you
- Access your current culture, does it fit with value-based care
- Culture "eats strategy" and unless you recognize what your culture is you cannot move forward
- A new culture will lead to success

For CPI:
- Keep on improving!

CONCLUSION

This is a most interesting time in our healthcare world! When the idea for this book was in its infancy, value-based, MACRA, prescription drug prices, were on the distant horizon. Much has changed in a short amount of time. We now have ABC, Amazon, Berkshire, and Chase headed by Atul Gawande, CVS merged, healthcare systems continuing to expand their footprint, CMS continuing to modify its approach to ACO's, major coding changes (E&M and telemedicine), greater need for cybersecurity. We are on a trajectory of change in healthcare.

But one thing doesn't change. It is up to the leadership and management of the medical practice to work together to OPTIMIZE the collective efforts to improve patient care. This can only be done by focusing on the issues, not getting lost in the maze of things happening, and keeping the focus on the patient.

It all starts with culture and strategy but as it has been said, culture trumps strategy. Simply put, the actions, words, focal points of activity, key expenditures, emphasis (or lack thereof) on patient care, communication, emphasis (or lack thereof) on learning, and the like will communicate to the practice team members what is important. This sets the framework for the future.

But no one person can do this alone. There needs to be relationships forged with all stakeholders in all points of the continuum of service and care. This is accomplished with a well-managed and financially stable organization. I wish you luck and let's improve healthcare together!

REFERENCES

1. https://www.dictionary.com/. Accessed December 1, 2018.
2. Gawande, A. *The Checklist Manifesto: How to Get Things Right*. Metropolitan Books-Macmillan, New York, NY. 2009.